THE ESSENTIALS OF INTERMITTENT FASTING FOR WOMEN 50 & BEYOND

A COMPREHENSIVE GUIDE TO WEIGHT LOSS, HORMONAL SUPPORT, AND HEALTHY AGING THROUGH FASTING

JESSICA CHRISTINE

Copyright © 2025 by Jessica Christine - All rights reserved.

The content within this book may not be reproduced, duplicated or transmitted without direct written permission from the author or the publisher.

Under no circumstances will any blame or legal responsibility be held against the publisher, or author, for any damages, reparation, or monetary loss due to the information contained within this book. Either directly or indirectly. You are responsible for your own choices, actions, and results.

Legal Notice:

This book is copyright-protected. This book is only for personal use. You cannot amend, distribute, sell, use, quote, or paraphrase any part, of the content within this book, without the consent of the author or publisher.

Disclaimer Notice:

Please note the information contained within this document is for educational and entertainment purposes only. All effort has been expended to present accurate, up-to-date, and reliable, complete information. No warranties of any kind are declared or implied. Readers acknowledge that the author is not engaging in the rendering of legal, financial, medical or professional advice. The content within this book has been derived from various sources. Please consult a licensed professional before attempting any techniques outlined in this book.

By reading this document, the reader agrees that under no circumstances is the author responsible for any losses, direct or indirect, which are incurred as a result of the use of the information contained within this document, including, but not limited to, — errors, omissions, or inaccuracies.

CONTENTS

Introduction	5
1. Understanding Intermittent Fasting	9
2. Crafting Your Personalized Fasting Plan	24
3. Nutrition and Meal Planning	37
4. Addressing Hormonal Changes and Health Concerns	50
5. Mental Clarity and Emotional Well-being	66
6. Overcoming Obstacles and Staying Motivated	78
7. Integrating Fasting with Holistic Health Practices	92
8. Scientific Insights and Future Perspectives	105
Conclusion	117
Book, Website & Podcast Recommendations	121
References	123

INTRODUCTION

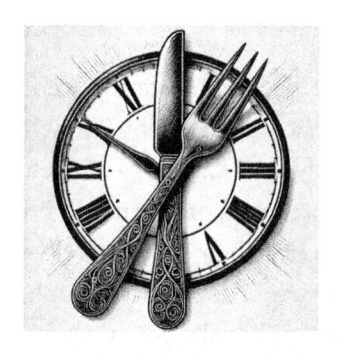

Reflecting on my life at 51, I find myself far from the dreams I once held. I don't have the "dream job," own a house, or possess the freedom to vacation at will. However, I am grateful for my health. Over the past few years, I unintentionally adopted a pattern of eating only during specific time frames. I gradually eliminated early breakfasts, began eating around lunchtime, and even incorporated 24-hour fasts once a month. Soon, I felt more energized and stronger. My weight decreased, and I avoided many common menopausal symptoms like hot flashes and brain fog. Unknowingly, I had embraced intermittent fasting. Intrigued, I delved deeper into the subject, which seamlessly aligned with my passion for nutrition. By doing so, it quickly became apparent that this information is vital for women my age. Many of my peers experience typical menopausal symptoms—some struggle with weight gain, while others endure night sweats that drench their beds. But this doesn't have to be our fate. We can change our narrative!

INTRODUCTION

Studies show that 60-70% of women aged 50 and above are overweight or obese, and many of us find ourselves battling the effects of menopause, such as brain fog, mood swings, and difficulty sleeping. It's a time in our lives when we often feel like our bodies are working against us despite our best efforts to maintain our health and vitality.

But what if I told you there's a scientifically proven way to reclaim control over your health and well-being? Intermittent fasting has emerged as a game-changer for women our age, offering a sustainable lifestyle solution that promotes weight loss and supports hormonal balance, mental clarity, and overall longevity.

As someone who has experienced the benefits of intermittent fasting firsthand, I've made it my mission to share this knowledge with other women who are ready to take charge of their health. With a comprehensive understanding of nutrition and a passion for empowering women to live their best lives, I've poured my expertise and personal experience into this book, creating an all-inclusive guide that will walk you through every step of your fasting journey.

Throughout these pages, you'll discover the science behind why intermittent fasting is so effective for women over 50, and you'll learn how to implement personalized fasting plans that fit seamlessly into your lifestyle. We'll explore the importance of nourishing your body with wholesome, nutrient-dense foods, and I'll share simple, delicious meal ideas that will make your fasting days a breeze. You'll find guidance on overcoming common obstacles, staying motivated, and incorporating gentle exercise routines to support your goals. Plus, you'll find a curated list of books, websites, and podcasts to motivate and elevate you on your journey.

INTRODUCTION

But more than just a how-to manual, this book is a source of empowerment and inspiration. I want you to know that you're not alone in this journey and that it's never too late to make positive changes in your life. By embracing intermittent fasting as a lifestyle rather than a temporary fix, you'll unlock a newfound sense of confidence, energy, and vitality that will radiate into every aspect of your being. Together, we'll dispel the myths surrounding intermittent fasting and show you how this ancient practice can be adapted to fit the unique needs of women our age.

Are you ready to embark on a transformative journey toward better health, hormonal balance, and a more vibrant self? Then, let's dive in together, one chapter at a time, as we unlock the essentials of intermittent fasting for women 50 and beyond. Your path to a healthier, happier you starts right here, right now.

1
UNDERSTANDING INTERMITTENT FASTING

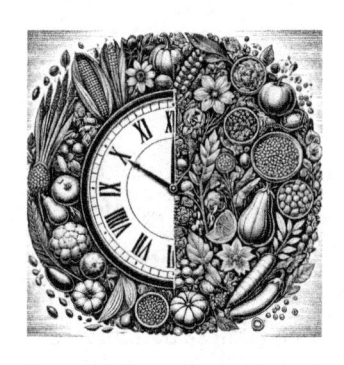

Have you ever stood in the kitchen, staring at the clock, wondering how you're supposed to fit yet another meal into your day? As women, particularly those over 50, we often find ourselves caught in a relentless cycle of eating schedules dictated by social norms rather than personal needs. And yet, here we are, seeking balance amidst the chaos of hormonal changes, fluctuating energy levels, and the constant battle with weight gain that seems to have settled like an unwelcome guest. I've engaged in numerous discussions with my peers on this topic, and there's an undeniable sense of frustration, often leading to a desire to surrender. However, with the adoption of intermittent fasting, it feels like a lifeline has been thrown into the sea of dietary confusion.

WHAT IS INTERMITTENT FASTING? A SIMPLE GUIDE

Intermittent fasting, at its core, is a pattern of eating that alternates between periods of fasting and eating. It's not about what you eat, but rather when you eat. It's a lifestyle choice that invites you to listen to your body's natural rhythms, allowing for periods of rest for your digestive system and, ultimately, for your entire body. This approach to eating is built around "eating windows" and "fasting periods." During an eating window, you consume all of your daily calories. The remaining time is spent fasting, during which only non-caloric beverages are typically consumed. For example, one might eat between 10 a.m. and 6 p.m., leaving the remaining 16 hours for fasting. This method, known as the 16:8 schedule, is the most popular and accessible for many. Alternatively, the 5:2 schedule involves eating normally for five days a week while reducing calorie intake to about 500-600 calories on the other two days. This flexibility allows you to tailor fasting to your lifestyle, making it a sustainable practice rather than a restrictive diet.

The beauty of intermittent fasting lies in its adaptability. One size does not fit all, and this approach respects that each of us has unique lifestyles and health goals. You can adjust your fasting and eating windows to suit your life, whether you're a retiree with leisurely mornings or a night owl who prefers late dinners. The timing isn't rigid but rather a guide to help you find what works best for your body. This flexibility extends beyond just the hours you choose to eat. It's about integrating fasting into your life in a way that enhances it, not restricts it. This is where the magic happens—it transforms from a diet to a lifestyle. When you embrace intermittent fasting, you're not

UNDERSTANDING INTERMITTENT FASTING

just making a temporary change but committing to a long-term shift that can bring profound benefits.

For women over 50, the benefits of intermittent fasting are particularly compelling. As we age, our bodies undergo changes that can make traditional dieting methods less effective. Metabolism slows, hormonal balance becomes more delicate, and maintaining energy levels can feel like an uphill battle. Intermittent fasting addresses these issues head-on. It supports weight management by promoting fat loss and preserving muscle mass. Many women report feeling more energetic and clear-headed, as fasting encourages mental clarity and sharpness. It also helps stabilize hormones, offering relief from the rollercoaster of menopause-related symptoms. And let's not overlook the digestive benefits; by giving your digestive system a break, you may experience improved gut health, less bloating, and a more comfortable relationship with food.

Intermittent fasting is not a fad. It's a sustainable lifestyle change that empowers you to take control of your health. It invites you to break free from the endless cycle of dieting and embrace a way of eating that supports your body's natural functions. You can redefine your relationship with food, to find joy in the freedom that comes from eating mindfully and living purposefully. As you embark on this path, remember that you are not alone. This book is here to guide you, offering support and encouragement each step of the way.

1.2 THE SCIENCE BEHIND FASTING: HOW IT AFFECTS YOUR BODY

The science of intermittent fasting is fascinating and empowering, offering us insights into how our bodies respond to periods of eating and fasting. At the heart of this process is ketosis, a metabolic state where the body shifts from using glucose as its primary energy source to burning stored fats. When we fast, glycogen stores in the liver deplete, prompting our bodies to use fat for fuel. This transition not only aids in weight loss but also contributes to a host of other health benefits, particularly for those of us navigating the challenges of midlife and beyond. It's akin to giving your body a tune-up, allowing it to run more efficiently by tapping into its energy reserves.

Another remarkable process that fasting activates is autophagy. This is the body's way of cleaning out damaged cells, making way for new, healthier ones. Think of it as a natural detoxification system that can enhance cellular repair and regeneration. During autophagy, cells break down and remove dysfunctional components, which can help protect against diseases linked to aging. The boost in cellular health is like a deep cleaning for your body, promoting longevity and resilience in ways that traditional diets often overlook.

Fasting also profoundly impacts insulin sensitivity. By reducing the frequency of insulin spikes, fasting helps our bodies become more responsive to insulin, lowering fasting glucose levels and reducing the risk of type 2 diabetes. This is particularly relevant for women over 50, as hormonal changes can affect insulin metabolism. Improved insulin sensitivity not only aids in weight management but also supports metabolic health, reducing the risk of chronic diseases that often accompany aging.

Regarding weight management, fasting offers a simple yet effective approach. By naturally reducing calorie intake, fasting can help create a caloric deficit, essential for weight loss.

UNDERSTANDING INTERMITTENT FASTING

Unlike restrictive diets that force us to count every calorie, fasting allows for a more intuitive relationship with food. It promotes fat burning by encouraging our bodies to access fat stores for energy, which can lead to more sustainable weight loss over time. This method aligns with the body's natural rhythms, making weight management feel less like a chore and more like a natural consequence of mindful eating.

The benefits extend beyond the physical, reaching into the realms of mental clarity and cognitive function. Fasting has been shown to enhance neuroplasticity, the brain's ability to form new neural connections. This is crucial for maintaining cognitive health as we age, supporting functions like memory and learning. Additionally, fasting increases the production of brain-derived neurotrophic factor (BDNF), a protein that plays a key role in brain health. Higher levels of BDNF are associated with improved mood and cognitive function, providing a mental boost that many find surprising and delightful.

Scientific research continues to support these benefits. Studies have demonstrated fasting's potential to improve metabolic markers, reduce inflammation, and even enhance longevity. According to a study published in *Nature* (2024), fasting affects major nutrient-sensing pathways, offering therapeutic potential for conditions ranging from cancer to neurodegeneration. Experts in nutrition and endocrinology have lauded fasting for its ability to promote health and well-being, particularly as a tool for managing the complexities of aging.

For women over 50, understanding these processes is empowering. It reframes fasting not just as a means to an end but as a holistic approach to health that respects and harnesses the body's innate wisdom. It's about working with your body, not against it, fostering an environment where you can thrive physically, mentally, and emotionally.

1.3 FASTING OVER 50: WHY IT'S DIFFERENT AND NECESSARY

As we age, our bodies undergo various changes that often feel relentless and challenging to manage. For women over 50, these changes can seem incredibly daunting. One of the most significant shifts is the slowing down of our metabolism, a process that seems to sneak up on us, making it harder to maintain a healthy weight. This metabolic slowdown means that the lifestyle choices that once kept us fit and healthy may no longer suffice. Coupled with this is the rollercoaster of hormonal fluctuations brought on by menopause, which can leave us feeling out of balance and out of sorts. These hormonal shifts are not just about hot flashes and mood swings; they also affect our energy levels, making it harder to muster the enthusiasm and vitality that once came so easily. Additionally, digestive issues can become more frequent, exacerbating the discomfort we feel in our bodies.

Brain fog is another common experience—a frustrating inability to think clearly or remember things as sharply as we once did. It's as if a cloud has settled over our minds, making simple tasks feel like monumental challenges. And then there's the seemingly inevitable weight gain, often settling around the abdomen, a stubborn visitor that refuses to leave despite our best efforts. These physiological changes are not just nuisances; they can significantly impact our quality of life and self-esteem.

Intermittent fasting offers a tailored approach to these issues, addressing them in a natural and effective way. For many women, fasting provides a way to manage weight gain specifically linked to post-menopausal changes. By allowing the body to burn fat more efficiently, fasting helps shed those extra pounds that seem immune to traditional dieting efforts. Beyond weight management, fasting supports bone health, which is an important consideration as we age and face increased risks of osteoporosis. It encourages the body to maintain bone density, safeguarding against fractures and other bone-related concerns.

Cognitive clarity is another remarkable benefit. By giving the brain a break from constant glucose processing, fasting can help clear the fog, enhancing mental acuity and focus. Women often report feeling a renewed sense of mental sharpness, a welcome change after years of struggling with forgetfulness and confusion. Energy levels, too, receive a boost. With fasting, the body learns to operate more efficiently, drawing on fat reserves for fuel and providing a steadier, more sustained energy supply. This means that those mid-afternoon slumps become less frequent, replaced by a consistent vitality that carries you through the day. One of the most significant advantages is the hormonal balance that fasting promotes. By stabilizing insulin and other hormone levels, fasting helps mitigate the tumultuous effects of menopause, offering relief from symptoms that can otherwise feel overwhelming.

It's crucial, however, to approach fasting with a personalized plan that considers your unique health profile. Women over 50 often have pre-existing health conditions that require careful consideration. Whether it's hypertension, diabetes, or another chronic issue, fasting can be adapted to suit your needs, ensuring that it supports rather than complicates your health. This may involve adjusting fasting times, incorporating specific supplements, or modifying exercise routines to align with your body's requirements. For instance, if you're on medication, timing your fasting periods around your dosage schedule can prevent any adverse effects. Incorporating gentle exercises, like yoga, jogging, or walking, can further enhance the benefits of fasting, keeping the body active without overexerting it.

Consider the story of Susan, a 55-year-old woman who felt trapped by her escalating weight and dwindling energy. She embraced intermittent fasting, tailoring it to her lifestyle and health needs. Over time, Susan shed the stubborn weight and woke up with more energy and a clearer mind. Her digestive issues subsided, and she experienced a level of control over her body that she hadn't felt in years. Susan's experience isn't unique; countless women have found similar success, each with their variations of fasting that fit their lives.

For instance, at 63, Roxanne struggled with gradual weight gain over two decades. After adopting intermittent fasting by limiting her eating to an 8-hour window between 11 AM and 7 PM, she lost 10 pounds in five months and felt more in control of her health.

Similarly, Laurie turned to intermittent fasting during menopause and noticed significant improvements in her energy levels and mental clarity within a week. Over time, she successfully lost weight and regained her vitality.

These examples highlight the potential benefits of intermittent fasting for women over 50 and emphasize the importance of personalizing the approach to individual lifestyles and health needs.

HORMONAL HEALTH AND FASTING: A SYMBIOTIC RELATIONSHIP

Navigating the maze of menopause can feel like trying to find your way through a fog with no map. The hormonal chaos accompanying this life stage often leaves us feeling out of sync with our bodies. This is where intermittent fasting steps in, offering a beacon of balance and control. Fasting influences our insulin levels, which are pivotal in managing blood sugar and energy. By reducing the frequency of insulin spikes, fasting helps to stabilize glucose levels, providing a more consistent energy flow and lessening the erratic highs and lows that can leave us feeling drained. This regulation helps mitigate the body's stress response, reducing cortisol levels, the hormone often responsible for overwhelming anxiety and stress.

For many women, the symptoms of menopause are a persistent reminder of the body's complex hormonal orchestra. Hot flashes, those unexpected waves of heat that seem to strike at the most inconvenient times, are a common complaint. So, too, are night sweats, which can disrupt sleep and leave you feeling exhausted before the day even begins. By promoting hormonal equilibrium, fasting can help reduce the frequency and intensity of these symptoms. It offers a measure of relief, allowing for a more stable mood and a greater sense of well-being. The impact on mood stability is particularly noteworthy. Fasting reduces cortisol and balances estrogen levels, and it can lead to improved emotional health, bringing a sense of calm and balance that feels like a breath of fresh air in the chaotic storm of menopause.

Fasting also supports metabolic health, a critical aspect of hormonal balance. Stabilizing blood sugar levels helps maintain a steady metabolic rate, which is crucial as we age. This stability reduces inflammation, a common contributor to chronic disease and general discomfort. Lower inflammation levels can improve cholesterol profiles, reducing the risk of heart disease and enhancing overall cardiovascular health. These metabolic benefits are not just about preventing disease; they're about improving the quality of life, allowing you to engage in daily activities more efficiently and with less pain.

To leverage fasting for hormonal balance, timing becomes a key player. Consider aligning your eating windows with your body's natural rhythms. Eating earlier in the day can support better glucose management and energy distribution. It's also essential to incorporate nutrient-rich foods during your eating periods. Focus on a diet rich in whole grains, plant proteins, and healthy fats. Foods like leafy greens, nuts, seeds, and tofu can provide the necessary nutrients to support hormone production and metabolic function. These choices nourish the body and support the intricate hormonal dance that keeps us balanced and well.

REFLECTION EXERCISE: UNDERSTANDING YOUR HORMONAL HEALTH

Please take a moment to reflect on how hormonal changes may influence your daily life. Keep a journal to gently track any symptoms, such as hot flashes, mood shifts, or changes in energy levels. Observing patterns related to your eating and fasting schedule can offer valuable insights into how your body responds. This practice is not about perfection but about understanding and supporting your body in the best way for you.

1.5 DEBUNKING MYTHS: COMMON MISCONCEPTIONS ABOUT FASTING

One of the most persistent myths surrounding intermittent fasting is the fear that it leads to muscle loss, particularly as we age. This concern, while understandable, is mainly unfounded when fasting is done correctly. During fasting periods, our bodies do not immediately start breaking down muscle for energy. Instead, they increase human growth hormone levels, which helps preserve lean muscle mass. The key to maintaining muscle while fasting lies in balancing periods of fasting with adequate nutrition and regular exercise. Consuming nutrient-rich foods during eating windows, particularly those high in protein, supports muscle maintenance. Engaging in resistance training or strength exercises further ensures your muscles remain strong and healthy. Just as a well-tuned orchestra requires all its instruments to play harmoniously, our bodies need nutrition and movement to keep muscle loss at bay.

Another common misconception is that fasting equates to starvation, a misunderstanding that can deter many from even considering it. There is a vast difference between controlled fasting and not eating at all. Fasting is a deliberate cycle of eating and resting, allowing your body to use stored energy efficiently. Adequate nutrition during eating windows is essential, ensuring your body receives the vitamins and minerals it needs to function optimally. While starvation deprives your body of vital nutrients, fasting provides a structured approach to eating that supports health without deprivation. The benefits of fasting—such as improved insulin sensitivity and reduced inflammation—far outweigh the risks when practiced thoughtfully and with attention to nutritional needs. It is akin to giving your body a well-deserved break, not punishing it through deprivation. The last thing we want is to spend the day feeling hungry. This shouldn't be the case when practicing intermittent fasting mindfully and intuitively.

Concerns about energy levels while fasting are also common, especially for those who lead busy lives. The notion that fasting leaves you sluggish and unproductive is quite the opposite of reality. Many individuals experience an increase in energy and alertness during fasting periods. This is because fasting improves energy balance by encouraging the body to use fat as a primary energy source, resulting in stable energy levels throughout the day. Furthermore, fasting can enhance cognitive function, improving focus and mental clarity. Tasks requiring attention and concentration become more manageable, not harder. The brain, often referred to as a powerhouse of energy, thrives on ketones produced during fasting, leading to sharper mental acuity and an overall sense of well-being.

Finally, there is the belief that fasting is unsuitable for older women, a misconception that undermines the very real benefits fasting can offer. Scientific research confirms that fasting is safe for older adults and offers several positive health outcomes. WebMD (2024) states, "Early studies show that it may also ward off certain muscle, nerve, and joint disorders that commonly affect women over 50." Research has demonstrated fasting's positive effects on metabolic health, longevity, and cognitive functions in older adults. Experts in gerontology and nutrition endorse fasting as a viable and effective strategy for managing the health challenges associated with aging. For women over 50, fasting can be a powerful tool to support health, providing a structured method to address age-related changes while enhancing quality of life. This endorsement from the scientific community provides reassurance that fasting is a safe and effective practice for those navigating this stage of life.

INTERMITTENT FASTING VS. TRADITIONAL DIETS: A COMPARATIVE INSIGHT

Through conversations with others who have tried various diets over the years, I noticed a common theme—traditional dieting often feels like an exhausting cycle of restriction. Counting calories, eliminating certain food groups, and constantly monitoring every bite creates a sense of scarcity. It is as if you are trapped in a cycle of temporary fixes, each promising quick results but failing to deliver sustainable change. Intermittent fasting, however, offers an entirely different approach. It's not about restricting what you eat; it's about when you eat. This shift from focusing on restriction to timing is a revelation. Allowing your body to rest between meals will enable it to use energy more efficiently, leading to a state of balance that is both achievable and sustainable.

The long-term sustainability of intermittent fasting sets it apart from traditional dieting. While diets often promise rapid weight loss, they rarely address the underlying behaviors and habits that lead to weight gain in the first place. Intermittent fasting, on the other hand, encourages a lifestyle change that is more about harmony than deprivation. Fasting offers a path to sustained health improvements instead of the short-lived results typical of conventional diets. It invites you to integrate habits that support well-being over the long haul rather than resorting to temporary measures that inevitably lead to yo-yo dieting. This sustainable approach is particularly beneficial for women over 50, as it aligns with the body's natural rhythms and needs.

One of the most profound psychological benefits of intermittent fasting is the healthier relationship it fosters with food. Dieting can often lead to an obsession with food, where every meal becomes a source of stress. Fasting alleviates this by reducing the frequency of meals, freeing you from constant preoccupation with what you can or cannot eat. This liberation allows you to enjoy food, savoring each bite without guilt or anxiety. With fasting, counting every calorie or obsessing over portion sizes is unnecessary. You learn to trust your body's hunger cues, creating a sense of empowering and refreshing freedom.

When comparing the effectiveness of fasting to traditional diets, the results speak for themselves. Studies have shown that fasting can lead to sustained weight loss and reduced body fat percentage. One such study titled: "Longer-term effects of intermittent fasting on body composition and cardiometabolic risk factors: A systematic review and meta-analysis" found that intermittent fasting (IF) significantly reduced body weight, body fat percentage, and fat mass. Specifically, compared to continuous calorie restriction (CR), IF led to a weighted mean difference (WMD) of -0.70 kg in fat mass and -0.59% in body fat percentage (Zou, Y., Zhang, Y., Zheng, L., & Zhu, J., 2023). Unlike many diets focusing solely on the scale, fasting also improves metabolic health by enhancing insulin sensitivity. This improvement in insulin function not only aids in weight management but also reduces the risk of metabolic diseases. The benefits extend beyond the physical, supporting mental and emotional health, which are often overlooked in diet culture. Fasting becomes more than a method of weight control; it's a holistic approach to wellness that nourishes both body and mind.

Fasting's role as a holistic lifestyle choice cannot be overstated. It seamlessly integrates into daily life, supporting mental, physical, and emotional health in a way few diets can. By aligning with your body's natural cycles, fasting promotes overall well-being, enhancing your quality of life on multiple levels. It's about finding balance and creating a lifestyle that supports all aspects of your health. The simplicity and adaptability of fasting make it an appealing choice for those seeking a comprehensive approach to health that doesn't sacrifice joy or freedom.

As I conclude this exploration of intermittent fasting, it's clear that this practice offers a pathway to health that is both empowering and sustainable. Unlike traditional diets, fasting frees you from the constraints of constant restriction, inviting you to embrace a balanced and mindful approach to eating. It supports your body's natural rhythms, fostering a relationship with food that is both nourishing and liberating. Whether seeking long-term weight management, improved metabolic health, or a more harmonious lifestyle, intermittent fasting offers a promising solution. Embrace the freedom it brings, and discover the lasting benefits of truly listening to your body's needs.

2

CRAFTING YOUR PERSONALIZED FASTING PLAN

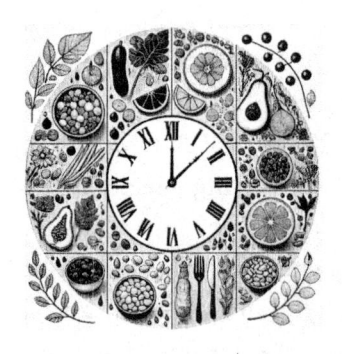

Women carry so many responsibilities that finding time for ourselves can feel nearly impossible. The demands on our schedules seem endless—like we're running on a treadmill that never slows down, repeating the same routine day after day. But at some point, we owe ourselves the opportunity to pause, reflect, and consider a different approach. Intermittent fasting offers not just a way to support our health but also an opportunity to reclaim time for ourselves. With so many fasting schedules, it's natural to feel unsure about where to start—but know that you're not alone in this journey, and there's a path that will work for you.

Choosing the proper fasting schedule is crucial, as it sets the foundation for success. Each fasting method has unique benefits and can be tailored to fit your lifestyle and goals. The 16:8 method, often considered the most balanced, involves fasting for 16 hours and eating during an 8-hour

CRAFTING YOUR PERSONALIZED FASTING PLAN

window. This schedule is ideal for maintaining energy levels and promoting gradual weight loss without drastically changing your daily routine. It works well for those with consistent daily schedules, offering structure without feeling restrictive.

On the other hand, the 20:4 schedule, also known as the Warrior Diet, is more intense. It involves a 20-hour fast and a 4-hour eating window. This method can benefit significant weight loss and those who prefer a more disciplined approach. It's challenging but rewarding for those who thrive on consistency and structure.

The 5:2 schedule offers another layer of flexibility, allowing for five days of regular eating and two non-consecutive days of reduced calorie intake, around 500-600 calories. This method is perfect for those who seek balance, providing the benefits of fasting without the commitment of daily practice. It's an excellent choice for anyone who enjoys socializing on weekends or has a variable schedule. Lastly, the eat-stop-eat method involves fasting for 24 hours once or twice a week. This periodic fasting can effectively break through weight loss plateaus, offering the body a reset while still allowing for flexibility throughout the week.

When considering which schedule might work best for you, evaluating your personal health goals is essential. If weight loss is a priority, a more intensive schedule like the 20:4 method might be appealing. The 16:8 schedule can provide stability without overwhelming changes for those seeking hormonal balance. Enhanced energy levels may be best achieved through a 5:2 schedule, allowing for regular eating most days while reaping the benefits of intermittent fasting. Mental clarity, a common goal for many, can often be improved with any fasting schedule, but finding the one that fits your life will amplify these benefits.

Understanding your lifestyle is key to selecting a fasting plan. Consider your work commitments and how fasting might fit into your daily schedule. If you work long hours or have unpredictable shifts, a flexible plan like the 5:2 method might work best, allowing you to structure fasting around your most manageable days. Social life is another factor; if dining out or family meals are frequent, you'll want a plan that accommodates these events without pressure or guilt. The beauty of fasting is its adaptability, allowing you to create a plan that feels like a natural part of your life rather than an imposition.

Consider the experience of Linda, a retiree who succeeded with the 16:8 method. After years of struggling with energy dips and weight gain, she discovered that this schedule provided the perfect structure. Linda enjoyed leisurely breakfasts and dinners with her partner, fitting her meals into an 8-hour window that aligned with her daily rhythm. Similarly, Janet, a caregiver for her elderly mother, benefitted from the 5:2 plan. With her unpredictable schedule, this method allowed Janet to focus on her responsibilities while prioritizing her health. She found that the flexibility of this schedule enabled her to maintain her energy and balance her caregiving duties with selfcare. These stories underscore the importance of choosing a fasting schedule that aligns with your life and goals.

CUSTOMIZING FASTING PLANS: FLEXIBILITY FOR EVERY LIFESTYLE

Life rarely fits neatly into a box, and neither should your fasting plan. As women, our days can be filled with unexpected events, whether a last-minute meeting, a family emergency, or

CRAFTING YOUR PERSONALIZED FASTING PLAN

simply an impromptu coffee date with a friend. Flexibility in fasting is crucial to accommodate these unpredictable elements without feeling like you're constantly breaking the rules. Adjusting your fasting windows for busy days is not about failing; it's about adapting your plan to suit your life. If you know an early breakfast meeting will disrupt your usual schedule, consider shifting your eating window slightly earlier or later. It's all about finding a rhythm that works for you, allowing your fasting plan to enhance your life, not hinder it.

When personalizing your fasting approach, consider what satisfies you within your eating windows. Incorporating your favorite foods can make the experience more enjoyable and sustainable. For instance, if you love starting your day with a hearty breakfast, adjust your fasting period to indulge in a morning meal. Conversely, if dinner is a cherished family time, let that be the focus of your eating window. The goal is to create a plan that feels like a natural extension of your lifestyle and preferences. Adjusting fasting periods to accommodate exercise routines is another way to tailor your plan. If your energy peaks in the afternoon and you prefer to exercise, consider scheduling your eating window to fuel your workouts and aid recovery.

Intuitive eating is an empowering principle that can complement fasting beautifully. It involves listening to your body's hunger cues during eating periods and balancing your food choices with nutritional needs. This means eating when you're hungry and stopping when you're satisfied, rather than by the clock or external rules. Pay attention to how different foods make you feel, and adjust your meals accordingly. Many women find that a protein-rich lunch helps them stay full longer, leading them to incorporate more of these foods into their diet. If that resonates with you, consider adding some excellent plant-based protein sources to your meals. Lentils, chickpeas, and black beans are rich in protein and fiber, supporting digestion and satiety. Quinoa is a nutrient-dense grain that provides all nine essential amino acids, making it a complete protein. Tofu, tempeh, and edamame are versatile, easy-to-digest options that can be included in various dishes. Nuts and seeds—such as almonds, chia seeds, flaxseeds, and hemp seeds—provide protein and offer healthy fats to nourish and satisfy you. For an extra boost, plant-based protein powders made from peas, hemp, or brown rice can help meet your protein needs. Dark leafy greens like spinach and kale, along with whole grains such as oats and farro, also contribute to your overall protein intake while delivering essential vitamins and minerals. Learning to eat intuitively encourages a mindful approach to food, helping you develop a deeper connection with your body's signals and needs.

REFLECTION SECTION: HONORING YOUR HUNGER

Take a few moments each day to gently tune into your hunger cues. Consider using a journal to note when you feel hungry and which foods genuinely nourish and satisfy you. With time, you'll gain a deeper understanding of your body's unique needs, allowing you to make fasting and eating choices that feel aligned and supportive of your well-being.

Consider Dina, a frequent traveler who found that flexibility in her fasting plan made all the difference. While initially skeptical about how fasting could fit into her hectic schedule, Dina discovered that she could maintain her health goals without stress by adjusting her fasting windows to accommodate flights and time zone changes. She learned to pack nourishing snacks for long flights and chose accommodations with kitchens so she could prepare meals. This adaptability made her feel in control, even when her environment constantly changed. Her story shows how minor adjustments can lead to significant success.

Ultimately, customizing your fasting plan is about making it work for you. There is no one-size-fits-all solution, and what works for one person might not work for another. Embrace the freedom to experiment and change your plan as needed. Remember, you are the author of your health story, and your fasting plan should reflect your unique lifestyle, preferences, and goals. By prioritizing flexibility and intuition, you can create a fasting approach that feels supportive and liberating, allowing you to thrive in all aspects of your life.

INCORPORATING FASTING WITH FAMILY MEALS

Navigating the complexities of family life while embracing intermittent fasting often feels like walking a tightrope. You're balancing your personal health goals with the need for harmonious family meals, a daily scenario many of us face. The challenge lies in coordinating meal times that accommodate your fasting schedule without disrupting the family's routine. It's common to encounter resistance from family members who aren't fasting, as they may not fully understand or support your choices. Managing diverse dietary preferences adds another layer of difficulty, especially if your family members have specific tastes or dietary restrictions. Picture the challenge of preparing just one meal that meets your nutritional needs while also pleasing everyone's tastes—it's no wonder it can feel overwhelming.

However, maintaining social connections during fasting does not need to be an exercise in frustration. It starts with communication. Sharing your fasting goals and their reasons with your family can foster understanding and support. Disclose how intermittent fasting supports your overall well-being and helps you align with your health goals. Planning shared meals within your eating windows is another practical strategy. This way, you can enjoy meals together without feeling like you're compromising on your fasting schedule. For instance, if your eating window begins at noon, plan a family brunch on weekends instead of breakfast. This slight adjustment can make a significant difference and allow everyone to participate in meal preparation and enjoyment.

Meal planning can be a powerful tool in successfully integrating fasting with family life. Consider introducing plant-based meal options that cater to everyone's taste while supporting your fasting goals. Dishes like hearty vegetable stews or quinoa salads are simple to prepare and packed with nutrients that benefit everyone. Another option is to focus on creating simple, nutritious dishes that can be customized to individual preferences. For example, taco nights can feature various fillings, allowing each family member to tailor their meal to their liking. By preparing versatile meals, you can accommodate your fasting needs while ensuring your family enjoys their favorites.

The story of Margaret, a grandmother who successfully integrated fasting with her family dinners, is particularly inspiring. She found herself in a predicament familiar to many: wanting to prioritize her health while remaining present in family life. By communicating her goals and involving her family in the process, Margaret managed to maintain her fasting schedule without missing out on cherished moments around the dinner

CRAFTING YOUR PERSONALIZED FASTING PLAN

table. She introduced family-friendly meals that fit her eating window, like roasted vegetable platters and whole grain pasta dishes, ensuring everyone was satisfied. Her family's support became a key factor in her success, allowing her to continue fasting without feeling isolated or deprived.

Balancing fasting with family meals doesn't have to be a solo endeavor. Involve your family in meal planning and preparation, making it collaborative. This not only eases the burden on you but also reinforces the idea that health and wellness are family values. It can be as simple as letting each family member choose a favorite dish to incorporate into the weekly menu, ensuring everyone feels included. As you navigate the intricacies of fasting within a family setting, remember that flexibility and open communication are your allies. By embracing these principles, you can create a supportive environment that honors your fasting goals and family traditions.

OVERCOMING INITIAL CHALLENGES: TIPS FOR BEGINNERS

Beginning intermittent fasting can feel like standing on the edge of a new adventure. Exciting, yet daunting. Many women encounter common hurdles, and it's essential to recognize these as part of the process. Initial hunger pangs often top the list. As your body adjusts to a new eating schedule, it's natural to feel hungry during fasting periods. This discomfort can sometimes lead to doubts about whether fasting is right for you. Another challenge is ensuring that meals are nutrient-dense, providing the energy and nourishment needed during eating windows. It requires a shift in mindset from focusing on quantity to quality, which may initially feel unfamiliar. Social pressure to eat can also be significant, especially in environments where food is a central component of social interactions. Whether it's a family gathering or a dinner with friends, the expectation to eat can challenge your commitment to fasting.

Fortunately, practical solutions exist to help you navigate these early difficulties. Starting gradually is one of the most effective strategies. Rather than diving into a full fasting schedule, begin with shorter fasting periods and gradually increase them as your body adapts. This approach eases you into the rhythm of fasting, making the transition smoother. Managing hunger involves listening to your body and finding what works best. Staying hydrated is crucial—we often confuse thirst with hunger, so drinking water or herbal teas can alleviate hunger. Engaging in light activities or distractions can also help shift focus away from hunger. Discussing your goals with family and social networks can provide a supportive environment. Sharing your reasons for fasting can foster understanding and reduce the pressure to eat during social occasions. Having allies who respect your choices can make a world of difference.

The psychological aspects of starting fasting are equally important. Overcoming food-related anxiety involves reframing how you view meals and food in general. It's about understanding that fasting isn't about deprivation but timing and balance. Social anxiety can also manifest, especially when others question your choices. This is where confidence in your decision comes into play. Acknowledging and addressing these mental barriers is key to successful fasting. It's a journey of not only physical change but also mental resilience. Shifting your mindset from scarcity to abundance can transform your relationship with food and fasting, turning challenges into opportunities for growth.

CRAFTING YOUR PERSONALIZED FASTING PLAN

To inspire and motivate, consider the words of renowned wellness expert Maya Angelou: "You may encounter many defeats, but you must not be defeated." This quote reminds us that initial setbacks don't define our fasting journey. They are simply stepping stones toward success. Take the story of Julia, who struggled through her first week of fasting. Faced with hunger and skepticism from those around her, she felt on the brink of giving up. But she persevered, leaning on her support network and focusing on her goals. By the end of the week, Julia noticed a shift—not just in her body but also in her mindset. She felt empowered and more in tune with her needs. Her experience underscores the importance of persistence and the rewards that follow when you stay committed to your health aspirations.

TRACKING YOUR PROGRESS: TOOLS AND TECHNIQUES

In the early days of intermittent fasting, it's completely natural to question whether you're making real progress. The mirror and the scale don't always reflect the whole picture, which can feel confusing or discouraging. This is where tracking can be beneficial. By documenting your journey, you can shift your focus beyond the day-to-day fluctuations and begin seeing the more profound, meaningful changes in your body and overall well-being. Today, technology offers a plethora of tools that can help you keep tabs on your fasting success. Fasting apps and digital journals have become invaluable allies for many, providing a convenient way to record fasting hours, meal plans, and even hydration levels. These apps often come with reminders, helping you maintain consistency and stay on track. Wearable fitness trackers add another layer, monitoring physical activity and sleep patterns and offering insights into how fasting affects overall wellbeing.

Keeping a fasting journal is more than just recording numbers; it becomes a personal narrative of growth and discovery. Documenting physical and emotional changes can provide motivation and clarity. You might write about how your energy levels fluctuate on different schedules or note mood changes and mental clarity changes. Tracking weight and measurements can give tangible evidence of progress, but remember, these numbers are just part of the story. Setting goals and achievements helps maintain focus, celebrating small victories along the way. This practice encourages reflection, allowing you to see patterns and make informed adjustments. It creates a personal record of your journey, offering encouragement on days when progress feels slow.

To evaluate the effectiveness of fasting, focus on metrics that truly matter. Energy levels provide immediate feedback on how fasting suits your body. Are you feeling more alert? Is that afternoon slump less pronounced? These shifts can be subtle yet significant. A reduction in glucose levels is another marker, indicating improved metabolic health. If you monitor these levels, note any changes and discuss them with your healthcare provider. Sleep quality is a crucial factor often overlooked. Better sleep can improve overall health and mood, a benefit frequently reported by those who fast. If you're experiencing fewer nighttime sweats or more restful sleep, these are signs that your body is responding positively.

Consider the story of Emily, who began her fasting journey feeling skeptical. She started using a simple app to log her fasting hours and soon noticed patterns she hadn't anticipated. By tracking her energy levels and sleep quality, she discovered that fasting improved her focus and reduced her anxiety. Emily also kept a journal where she noted emotional breakthroughs and occasional setbacks. This documentation process became a source of inspiration, showing her progress beyond what the scale reflected. Emily's example illustrates how tracking can transform abstract feelings into concrete evidence, reinforcing your commitment and guiding your path.

ADJUSTING YOUR PLAN: HOW TO TWEAK FOR BETTER RESULTS

Life is a constant ebb and flow, and so should be your approach to intermittent fasting. Recognizing when your fasting plan needs adjustment as your body and lifestyle evolve is vital. Changes in your energy levels, mood swings, or even small weight fluctuations can signal that it's time to rethink your strategy. For instance, if you feel excessively fatigued or unable to focus, these might be cues from your body asking for a tweak in your fasting schedule or nutritional intake. This is where giving yourself grace becomes essential. Adjustments are not failures but a testament to your commitment to listening to and respecting your body's needs. Your body is your best guide—you'll know how to move forward when you hear it.

Consider shortening or lengthening your fasting periods to better align with your current lifestyle. A longer eating window may provide flexibility if your mornings have become more hectic. Alternatively, if you're experiencing late-night cravings, extending your fasting period could help curb those urges. Experimenting with meal compositions during your eating window can also make a significant difference. Introduce more nutrient-dense foods or adjust your macronutrient balance to see how your body responds. Sometimes, a slight protein or fiber intake shift can improve satiety and energy levels. It's about finding the combination that leaves you feeling nourished and energized.

Feedback is crucial in refining your fasting approach. Regularly reassessing your goals can provide clarity and direction. Are you still striving for weight loss, or has your focus shifted to maintaining energy throughout the day? These reflections can inform necessary adjustments to your plan.

Imagine the story of Laura, who felt drained halfway through her workday. Through feedback and self-reflection, she discovered that her body thrived with a slightly earlier eating window. By adjusting her schedule, Laura improved her energy and noticed a newfound mental clarity that enhanced her productivity. Her experience highlights the importance of being attuned to your body's signals and being open to change.

As you explore what works best for you, remember that your fasting plan is a living, breathing entity. It should evolve with you, reflecting your current needs and aspirations. Embrace this adaptability as a strength, not a weakness. By staying responsive to your body and remaining open to adjustments, you create a sustainable and fulfilling fasting experience that empowers you to live your best life.

This chapter reminds us that intermittent fasting is not a one-size-fits-all endeavor. It's a personalized approach that requires continual adaptation and mindfulness. As you move forward, embrace the flexibility and insights gained from your journey, knowing that each adjustment brings you closer to a plan that genuinely supports your well-being and lifestyle.

3
NUTRITION AND MEAL PLANNING

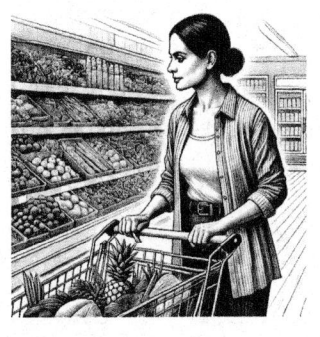

Picture this: a vibrant farmer's market bustling with life, the air filled with the earthy aroma of fresh produce. You weave through the stalls, marveling at the kaleidoscope of fruits and vegetables, each one more enticing than the last. It's here, amidst the kale and berries, that the journey to nutrient-dense eating begins. As women over 50, our nutritional needs evolve, demanding foods that fill us up and fuel our bodies with the essential nutrients needed for vibrant health. Nutrient density becomes the cornerstone of our meal planning, offering a path to meet our fasting goals and thrive.

When you think of nutrient-dense foods, envision leafy greens like spinach, kale, and Swiss chard. These powerhouses contain vitamins A, C, and K and essential minerals like calcium and iron. Cruciferous vegetables such as broccoli and brussels sprouts offer a similar bounty, supporting your immune system and aiding in hormonal balance. With their rich array of antioxidants, berries are perfect for reducing oxidative stress—a key factor in aging. Whether you sprinkle them on your morning oatmeal or blend them into a smoothie, these fruits help protect your cells from damage, offering a delicious and easy way to incorporate vital nutrients into your diet.

Consider beans and legumes for plant proteins. They provide a double dose of fiber and protein, keeping you full and satisfied while supporting muscle maintenance. Lentils, chickpeas, and black beans are versatile additions to salads, soups, and stews, transforming simple dishes into nutrient-rich meals. The importance of these foods cannot be overstated, especially as we look to maintain muscle mass and manage weight. The fiber content aids digestion, ensuring our nutrients are absorbed efficiently, reducing bloating, and enhancing gut health.

As we age, certain nutrients become particularly crucial. Calcium takes center stage, with its role in maintaining bone health. Women over 50 require about 1,200 mg daily to combat the risk of osteoporosis. Incorporate calcium-rich foods like fortified plant milks, tofu, almonds, and leafy greens into your meals. Omega-3 fatty acids in flaxseeds, chia seeds, and walnuts support heart health and cognitive function. These essential fats help reduce inflammation, lowering the risk of chronic diseases. Whole grains, fruits, and vegetables should fill your plate, offering a rainbow of nutrients that support every aspect of your health.

Incorporating these nutrient-dense foods into your meals can be simple and rewarding. Embrace their diverse textures and flavors, and your meals will nourish your body and bring joy and satisfaction to your eating experience.

NUTRITION AND MEAL PLANNING

There's something truly special about seasonal and locally grown produce. Choosing ingredients that grow harmoniously with nature nourishes your body and supports local farmers and sustainable agriculture. Seasonal fruits and vegetables are often richer in flavor and nutrients, harvested at their peak for maximum freshness and health benefits. Visiting your local farmers' market can be a delightful experience—let the vibrant colors and fresh aromas inspire your choices. Beyond just a meal, this simple act fosters a deeper connection to your food, community, and the land that sustains us.

REFLECTION ACTIVITY: BUILDING YOUR NUTRIENT-RICH PLATE

Close your eyes for a moment and picture your ideal meal. What colors pop from the plate? What textures excite your senses? What flavors make your mouth water? Let this vision guide your next shopping trip, filling your basket with vibrant, nutrient-dense foods that nourish you. As you choose each ingredient, consider how it supports your health and well-being. Then, have fun experimenting with new recipes that bring your plate and energy to life. To deepen the experience, keep a journal to reflect on how these changes make you feel physically and emotionally.

Intermittent fasting is not just about when you eat but what you eat. Focusing on nutrient-dense foods empowers your body to function at its best, supporting your fasting goals with the vitality needed to navigate life's beautiful complexities.

PLANT-BASED MEALS: SIMPLE RECIPES FOR EVERY PALATE

Transitioning to a plant-based diet can feel like a leap into the unknown, yet the benefits are profound. By focusing on plant-based meals, you enhance the fasting benefits and support your overall health in innovative and nurturing ways. Plant-based eating can significantly improve digestion and gut health, thanks to the high fiber in fruits, vegetables, and legumes. This fiber acts like a gentle broom, sweeping through your digestive tract, promoting regularity, and reducing bloating. Additionally, embracing a plant-based lifestyle supports heart health by lowering cholesterol and blood pressure levels and reducing the risk of chronic diseases such as diabetes and cancer. In fact, The Atherosclerosis Risk in Communities (ARIC) Study, starting in 1985 -ongoing, has found that "diets higher in plant foods were significantly associated with a reduced risk of cardiovascular disease, cardiovascular mortality, and all-cause mortality" (Journal of the American Heart Association, 2019). As you fill your plate with colorful produce, you also engage in better weight management. Plant-based meals tend to be lower in calories yet high in nutrients, allowing you to nourish your body without excess. Enhanced brain function is another delightful benefit, as the antioxidants and healthy fats found in plants contribute to cognitive health. Moreover, a plant-rich diet reduces inflammation, is a silent contributor to many ailments, and supports longevity, enabling you to live life with energy and enthusiasm.

Incorporating plant-based meals into your routine doesn't have to be complicated or time-consuming. Consider starting with a quinoa and black bean salad. Simply cook quinoa, toss it with black beans, diced bell peppers, corn, and fresh cilantro,

NUTRITION AND MEAL PLANNING

and dress it with lime juice and a sprinkle of olive oil. It's refreshing, filling, and packed with protein and fiber. A lentil soup with seasonal vegetables offers warmth and nutrition for cooler days. Simmer lentils with carrots, celery, tomatoes, and herbs for a comforting dish that satisfies the palate and the soul. A chickpea stir-fry is another quick option, combining chickpeas with broccoli, bell peppers, and a savory sauce of soy and sesame oil. For something heartier, try a butternut squash lasagna, layering roasted squash with spinach and a creamy cashew sauce between whole-grain noodles. These recipes cater to all tastes, offering a blend of flavors and textures that make each meal an experience to savor.

When transitioning to more plant-based meals, replace animal protein with plant protein. Incorporate lentils, chickpeas, seitan, and tofu into your dishes, allowing these versatile proteins to become the star of your meals. Experiment with meatless days, dedicating certain days of the week to plant-based eating. This approach eases the transition and introduces variety and excitement into your culinary routine. These plant-based meals leave you feeling more energized and satisfied. As you explore new ingredients and flavors, you'll discover a world of culinary possibilities that enrich your dining experience while supporting your health goals.

Consider the story of Abby, who embraced plant-based eating and experienced a remarkable increase in energy. Her mornings became brighter and invigorating, with a newfound zest for her daily activities. Her digestion improved, and she no longer felt the discomfort that had plagued her for years. Catherine, another woman who shifted to a plant-focused diet, reversed her diabetes diagnosis. By eliminating processed foods and focusing on whole, plant-based ingredients, Catherine regained control over her health, finding empowerment in her food choices. These testimonials highlight the transformative impact of plant-based eating, inspiring and empowering those striving for a healthier, more vibrant life.

MEAL TIMING AND ITS IMPACT ON FASTING SUCCESS

Picture yourself at the start of a busy day, juggling responsibilities and maintaining the delicate balance between your commitments and personal well-being. Amid this whirlwind, the timing of your meals can play a pivotal role in managing your energy and overall health. Meal timing during intermittent fasting is not just about the hours you choose to eat; it's about aligning those hours with your body's natural rhythms to optimize metabolic health. It's about finding the sweet spot where your energy levels peak and your body processes nutrients most efficiently. Timing meals to coincide with your circadian rhythms can enhance these benefits, as research suggests that our bodies are more insulin-sensitive earlier in the day (WebMD, 2024). By consuming your largest meal in the morning or early afternoon, you support your metabolism in a way that aligns with your body's biological clock. This practice enhances energy levels and helps maintain metabolic stability, setting the stage for a productive day.

Planning meal timing strategically can significantly influence the success of your fasting regimen. Eating your largest meal earlier in the day takes advantage of the body's heightened metabolic capacity, promoting better digestion and nutrient absorption. Consistency is key, as regular mealtimes help regulate internal clocks that govern hormone production and digestion. This consistency aids in maintaining stable energy levels and metabolic health, reducing the likelihood of mid-

NUTRITION AND MEAL PLANNING

afternoon slumps. However, life is rarely predictable, and challenges to maintaining ideal meal schedules will arise. Social gatherings, for instance, can disrupt your routine. One solution is to adjust your fasting window slightly on these days, allowing for participation without guilt. Managing hunger and cravings during fasting periods is another common obstacle. Staying hydrated is crucial, as dehydration can often be mistaken for hunger. Keep a bottle of water or herbal tea handy to sip throughout the day, helping fend off cravings and maintaining focus.

Consider the story of Elaine, who found that adjusting her meal timing improved her fasting success and her sleep quality. She noticed deeper, more restful sleep by shifting her eating window to end earlier in the evening. This simple change allowed her body to wind down naturally, free from the burden of late-night digestion. Her mornings became a time of clarity and energy, a transformation that highlighted the profound impact of meal timing on overall well-being. Another example is Linda, who experienced a boost in energy through strategic meal planning. By front-loading her meals and focusing on nutrient-dense options in the morning, Linda felt sustained energy throughout the day, allowing her to engage fully with her daily activities without frequent snacks or caffeine boosts. These examples showcase how mindful meal timing can transform fasting from a mere schedule into a seamless, harmonious part of your lifestyle.

BALANCING MACRONUTRIENTS: CARBS, PROTEINS, AND FATS

Imagine sitting down to a beautifully balanced meal, each element working harmoniously to nourish your body and mind. This is the power of balancing macronutrients: the dance of carbohydrates, proteins, and fats that form the foundation of a healthy diet. As women over 50, our bodies rely on this balance to maintain energy, support muscle health, and keep our brains sharp. Proteins are the building blocks crucial for muscle maintenance. They help repair tissues and support a robust metabolism. As we age, preserving muscle mass becomes more important, and ensuring adequate protein intake can significantly affect how we feel and function. Think of proteins as the scaffolding that keeps us strong and resilient, especially during fasting periods when our bodies may tap into muscle stores if protein intake is insufficient.

Proteins aren't the only key players. Healthy fats are equally vital, acting as the brain's best friend. These fats in foods like avocados, olive oil, and nuts provide essential fatty acids that support cognitive health. They also play a role in hormone production and maintaining cell structure. Fats are the long-burning fuel that keeps you going, offering sustained energy and helping you feel satisfied after meals. They slow digestion, allowing for the gradual release of glucose into the bloodstream, preventing energy crashes and keeping you feeling full longer.

Carbohydrates, often misunderstood, are necessary for energy. They are the body's preferred fuel source, especially for the brain and during physical activity. The key is to focus on complex carbohydrates, like whole grains, legumes, and vegetables, which provide a steady energy supply without rapid spikes in blood sugar levels. These carbs are packed with fiber, supporting digestion and promoting feelings of fullness. They are the steady beat in your body's symphony, keeping everything in sync and functioning smoothly.

When distributing these macronutrients, consider aiming for a meal composition of about 40% carbohydrates, 30% protein, and 30% fats. This ratio supports balanced energy levels and overall health, aligning with the needs of a woman over 50. Incorporating plant protein sources like tofu, tempeh, and lentils supports muscle health and offers a wealth of vitamins and minerals that enhance well-being. Including various protein sources ensures you get a range of essential amino acids, supporting the body's diverse needs.

The impact of these macronutrient choices on energy and satiety is profound. High-protein meals, for instance, increase feelings of fullness, reducing the likelihood of overeating later in the day. This is particularly beneficial during fasting, where maintaining satiety can help manage hunger during fasting windows. Healthy fats, on the other hand, provide that steady, slow-burning energy that keeps you alert and focused, whether you're tackling a busy workday or enjoying a leisurely afternoon. They are the key to prolonged energy, preventing the peaks and valleys that can make fasting challenging.

For meal ideas that showcase balanced macronutrient distribution, consider dishes like grilled tofu with quinoa and steamed vegetables. This satisfying meal offers a mix of protein, complex carbohydrates, and healthy fats, providing everything your body needs to thrive. Another option is soy yogurt with mixed berries and almonds, which delivers protein, fiber, and healthy fats in a delicious, easy-to-prepare breakfast or snack. These meals illustrate how balance can be both nourishing and satisfying, supporting your fasting goals while keeping you energized and content.

THE ROLE OF HYDRATION: STAYING WELL-HYDRATED

Imagine waking up each morning feeling as though you've been quenched from the inside out, ready to take on whatever the day has in store. Staying well-hydrated plays a pivotal role in achieving this feeling, especially when you're embracing intermittent fasting. Hydration is not merely a matter of quenching thirst; it's a fundamental aspect of supporting your body's myriad functions. When fasting, your body isn't taking in calories but still requires water to maintain its processes. Proper hydration can prevent the fatigue often associated with dehydration, making fasting periods feel more grueling than needed. Additionally, staying hydrated aids in detoxification processes, helping your body flush out toxins and maintain balance. It's like giving your body a fresh start each day, ensuring all systems run smoothly.

To maintain hydration during fasting, consider starting your day with a glass of water upon waking up. This simple act kick-starts your metabolism and prepares your body for the day ahead. Incorporating herbal teas and infusions throughout the day can provide a comforting and varied way to stay hydrated. Herbal teas like chamomile or peppermint can also have calming effects, an added bonus during fasting days. It's essential to avoid sugary or highly caffeinated drinks, as they can lead to dehydration and disrupt your fasting goals. Instead, choose water-rich beverages that hydrate without adding unnecessary calories or causing energy spikes and crashes.

Hydrating foods can also be essential in maintaining your fluid balance, especially during eating windows. Foods like cucumbers, oranges, and watermelon are refreshing and packed with

NUTRITION AND MEAL PLANNING

water, making them ideal snacks during your eating periods. Soups and broths, rich in nutrients and hydration, can be a warming and satisfying choice, particularly in cooler weather. These foods provide a dual benefit, nourishing your body while boosting your hydration levels. They're easy to incorporate into your meals, offering versatility and balance to your diet.

Women prioritizing hydration often share remarkable improvements in their health and fasting experience. Take, for example, an old colleague I know who started her fasting journey feeling sluggish and mentally foggy. By staying hydrated, Kathy noticed a significant increase in her energy levels and mental clarity. She described feeling more awake and engaged throughout the day, her thoughts flowing more freely as if a weight had been lifted. Kathy's testimony is a powerful reminder of how something as simple as adequate hydration can dramatically enhance your well-being, making fasting achievable and enjoyable.

SUPPLEMENTS AND FASTING: WHAT TO CONSIDER

Navigating the world of supplements can feel like walking through a labyrinth. Determining what's beneficial and unnecessary can be overwhelming, with so many options. Yet, as women over 50, we face unique nutritional needs that sometimes require a little extra support. This is where supplements come in, offering a way to fill those gaps and enhance overall well-being. Supplements can act as a safety net, ensuring you receive the nutrients your body needs to thrive, mainly when dietary intake might not cover all bases. They help bolster nutritional reserves, supporting everything from bone health to metabolic function, which is crucial as we navigate the changes that come with age.

Selecting the right supplements requires careful consideration and guidance. It's important to consult healthcare professionals before introducing any supplement into your regimen. They can provide personalized advice based on your medical history, current health status, and specific needs. This step is crucial in ensuring that any supplement you choose will benefit rather than harm you. When browsing through the myriad of options available, prioritize whole-food-based supplements. These are often more bioavailable, meaning your body can absorb and utilize them more effectively. Supplements derived from whole foods tend to provide a complex array of nutrients, mirroring the diversity found in nature. This holistic approach particularly benefits those looking to support their body's intricate systems.

Certain supplements are highly recommended for many women over 50. Vitamin D is often at the top of the list. It supports bone health by aiding calcium absorption. Maintaining bone density becomes increasingly vital as we age, and vitamin D plays a pivotal role in this process. Magnesium is another supplement worth considering. It supports muscle and nerve function, helping to prevent cramps and spasms that can sometimes accompany fasting. Additionally, magnesium regulates sleep patterns, promoting better rest and recovery. While these supplements are beneficial, they are not a one-size-fits-all solution. They should be tailored to your unique health profile and needs, complementing your fasting lifestyle without causing imbalances.

However, supplements must be approached with care, as they can interact with medications in ways that may alter their effectiveness or cause unintended side effects. This highlights the need for personalized medical guidance to ensure safety and compatibility. Regularly monitoring for any changes in how you feel and adjusting your supplement regimen as needed is key to maintaining a balanced, health-conscious approach. By staying mindful and informed, you can ensure that supplements support your well-being without unintended consequences.

As we conclude this nutrition and meal-planning chapter, remember that supplements are just one piece of the wellness puzzle. They support a foundation of nutrient-dense foods, plant-based meals, and mindful meal timing. Together, these elements create a holistic approach to health, empowering you to navigate fasting with confidence and vitality. In the next chapter, we'll explore how intermittent fasting can address hormonal changes and health concerns unique to women over 50, continuing our journey toward optimal health and well-being.

4
ADDRESSING HORMONAL CHANGES AND HEALTH CONCERNS

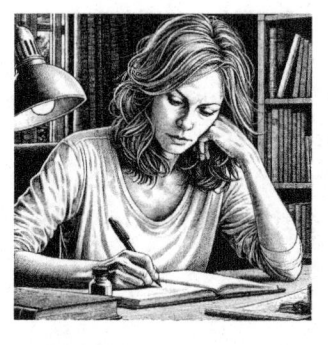

For many women our age, menopause can feel like an uninvited guest, arriving with changes that may challenge even the most resilient among us. It marks a significant transition, affecting our bodies in ways that can be both puzzling and difficult to navigate. As estrogen levels drop, many women experience a slowdown in metabolic rate, a change that impacts everything from energy levels to the way our bodies store fat. This hormonal shift is accompanied by changes in fat distribution, often leading to increased abdominal adiposity—the medical term for that stubborn belly fat that seems immune to our efforts. This redistribution of fat alters our physical appearance and affects our metabolic health, contributing to conditions like insulin resistance and even metabolic syndrome (Prevention, 2024). These changes can feel overwhelming, leaving us searching for solutions that align with our new reality.

Intermittent fasting emerges as a beacon of hope amidst these challenges, offering a method that harmonizes with the body's natural rhythms. By embracing fasting, you can positively influence metabolic health in profound ways. One of the key benefits is regulating blood sugar levels, which helps stabilize energy and mood. Fasting encourages the body to use stored fat for fuel, a process known as enhanced fat oxidation. This not only aids in weight management but also reduces the risk of developing type 2 diabetes, a concern that grows more pressing as we age. Fasting's ability to lower insulin levels further supports this process, creating a metabolic environment that promotes health rather than hinders it.

The scientific community has recognized fasting's impact on metabolic health, with research highlighting its benefits for menopausal women. Research has shown that intermittent fasting can improve metabolic rate (Nature, 2024), helping to counteract the natural slowdown associated with menopause. Endocrinologists often support fasting as a viable strategy for managing these changes, citing its ability to enhance insulin sensitivity and support fat metabolism. These expert insights provide reassurance that fasting is not just a trend but a grounded approach to health that acknowledges the unique challenges faced by women over 50.

Incorporating fasting into your lifestyle requires a mindful and gradual approach, especially during menopause. Ease into it by starting with shorter fasting periods, giving your body time to adapt before gradually extending the window. Staying well-hydrated is essential, as water supports vital functions and helps curb hunger during fasting. Complementing fasting with resistance training can further enhance its benefits by preserving muscle mass and supporting metabolic health. Even light strength exercises help counteract the natural decline in muscle that comes with age. Additionally, integrating yoga and meditation can promote flexibility, reduce stress, and cultivate a sense of physical and mental balance.

Another key strategy is timing meals to optimize metabolism. Consider aligning your eating windows with your body's natural energy peaks, typically earlier in the day. This alignment supports insulin sensitivity and can lead to more stable energy levels throughout the day. By consuming nutrient-dense meals that balance carbohydrates, proteins, and healthy fats, your body has the fuel it needs to thrive. These steps, while simple, create a foundation for metabolic health that supports your body's needs during menopause and beyond.

Reflect on your experiences and consider how fasting might fit into your life's tapestry. As you embark on this chapter of your journey, know that you are supported by a community of women who share your struggles and triumphs. Together, we navigate the complexities of hormonal changes armed with knowledge and resilience, ready to embrace the health and vitality that intermittent fasting can bring.

MANAGING HOT FLASHES AND MOOD SWINGS WITH FASTING

My friends and I have had countless conversations about menopause—it's a topic that never seems to run out of new surprises. When you're in the thick of it, it can feel like your body has become a stranger overnight. Hot flashes barge in uninvited, striking at the worst possible moments, leaving you flushed and frustrated. And then there are the mood swings—like an unpredictable rollercoaster you never signed up for, taking you on a wild ride of emotions without warning. These symptoms are not random; they stem from our bodies' intricate dance of hormones. As we age, fluctuations in estrogen and progesterone disrupt the balance that once seemed so effortless. The hypothalamus, the part of the brain responsible for regulating body temperature, becomes particularly sensitive to these changes. It misinterprets minor variations in temperature as overheating, triggering hot flashes. Meanwhile, mood swings arise from the same hormonal imbalances, affecting neurotransmitters that regulate mood and emotion.

Intermittent fasting offers a potential pathway to stability amidst this hormonal chaos. By adopting a fasting regimen, you may find relief from these symptoms, as fasting helps stabilize hormone levels. One of the ways it achieves this is by regulating insulin levels, a hormone closely linked to energy and mood. As insulin levels stabilize, the body experiences less fluctuation in blood sugar, leading to steadier energy levels throughout the day. Furthermore, fasting reduces cortisol production, the stress hormone that can exacerbate feelings of anxiety and stress. Lower cortisol levels contribute to a calmer, more balanced emotional state, making mood swings less severe and frequent. These changes promise a more serene and predictable daily experience, allowing you to navigate menopause with greater ease and confidence.

In sharing the stories of other women, I find encouragement and hope. Take Erin, for example, a friend who struggled with intense hot flashes that disrupted her sleep and daily life. After incorporating fasting into her routine, she noticed a significant decrease in their frequency and intensity. Her nights became more restful, and her days were no longer marked by the anxiety of anticipating the next wave of heat. Her personal story, though anecdotal, provides a glimpse into the potential that fasting holds for managing menopausal symptoms, reminding us that change is possible and that we are not alone in our struggles.

Dietary choices also play a crucial role in managing these symptoms. Incorporating foods rich in phytoestrogens, like flaxseeds, soy products, and legumes, can support hormonal balance. Phytoestrogens mimic estrogen in the body, providing a gentle boost to levels that may have dropped. Cruciferous vegetables, such as broccoli, cauliflower, and brussels sprouts, are another excellent addition to your diet. They contain compounds that help metabolize estrogen, aiding in hormonal regulation. Seeds rich in omega-3 fatty acids, including chia seeds, flaxseeds, and walnuts, support overall brain health and may help stabilize mood. These healthy fats contribute to brain function, reducing inflammation and promoting emotional well-being. On the other hand, be mindful of foods and drinks that can trigger or worsen symptoms. Caffeine and spicy foods, for example, are well-known culprits that can intensify hot flashes and disrupt sleep. By making thoughtful dietary choices, you can create a more balanced and supportive environment for your body, helping to ease discomfort and promote overall well-being.

REFLECTION SECTION: EXPLORING YOUR TRIGGERS

Pause for a moment and think about your experiences with hot flashes and mood swings. Have you noticed any patterns? Remember that keeping a journal can be a powerful tool to track when these symptoms arise and what you ate or did beforehand. Over time, you may start to uncover hidden triggers, helping you make more informed choices about your diet and lifestyle. By tuning into your body's responses, you can make adjustments that bring greater balance, comfort, and well-being.

BOOSTING ENERGY LEVELS: FASTING FOR VITALITY

At our age, fatigue becomes a typical unwelcome companion and familiar adversary, often rooted in slowed metabolism, nutrient deficiencies, and lack of sleep. Our bodies no longer process nutrients with the same efficiency they once did, and this metabolic sluggishness can leave us feeling drained. Emotional stress compounds the issue, leaving us longing for the energy of our youth. With the weight of these factors, it's easy to feel overwhelmed and resigned to a life of perpetual tiredness. However, intermittent fasting offers an intriguing solution that is the key to reclaiming the elusive energy.

Fasting can naturally boost your energy levels in several ways. On a cellular level, it helps your mitochondria—the tiny power plants of your cells—work more efficiently. These mitochondria produce the energy your body needs, and when you fast, they become better at generating energy while creating less waste. This means your body can sustain energy levels more effectively throughout the day. As a result, tasks that once felt draining may start to feel more manageable, as your body learns to tap into its energy reserves more efficiently. This isn't just a quick boost—it's a long-term shift in how your body fuels itself, providing more steady and reliable energy.

The stories of women who have experienced increased vitality through fasting are inspiring and illuminating. Take the case of Patricia, who had long struggled with afternoon fatigue that seemed to sap her productivity and joy. After incorporating fasting into her routine, she noticed a marked improvement in her stamina. She no longer needed a post-lunch nap to function, and her afternoons became a time of productivity rather than rest. Testimonials like hers showcase the power of fasting to revitalize energy levels, offering a glimpse into life without the constant weight of fatigue.

Consider adopting supportive habits and routines to maintain steady energy levels while fasting. Regular physical activity plays a key role in energy management, improving circulation, and enhancing mood. During fasting periods, choose gentle exercises like yoga or walking to stay active without overexerting yourself while saving more intense workouts for your eating windows when your energy stores are replenished. Nutrition is just as important—ensuring a balanced protein intake, healthy fats, and carbohydrates during your eating periods helps sustain energy throughout the day. Additionally, managing stress is essential, as chronic stress can be a significant drain on vitality. Mindfulness practices like meditation and breathwork can help you stay calm, focused, and energized.

Quality sleep is another vital component of managing energy levels. Prioritizing restful sleep allows your body to recharge fully, setting the stage for a day filled with energy and clarity. Establish a bedtime routine promoting relaxation, such as reading or a warm bath. Aim to maintain a consistent sleep schedule by going to bed and waking up at the same time each day. Reducing screen time before bed can also enhance sleep quality, allowing you to wake refreshed and ready to embrace the day. When combined, these practices create a supportive environment for fasting, enabling you to fully harness its energy-boosting potential and step into each day with renewed vigor.

ADDRESSING HORMONAL CHANGES AND HEALTH CONC...

WEIGHT MANAGEMENT: COMBATING STUBBORN WEIGHT GAIN

In the years following menopause, many women find themselves grappling with weight gain that seems to defy their every effort. This challenge isn't just about a few extra pounds; it's about the frustrating shift in how our bodies store fat. As estrogen levels decline, there is a significant increase in abdominal fat, a shift that often feels beyond our control. This change is coupled with a naturally slower metabolic rate, making it even more difficult to shed unwanted weight. The impact of these hormonal changes is profound, often leaving us feeling as if we're fighting an uphill battle against our biology. Seeing the scale climb despite healthy eating and regular exercise can be disheartening, particularly when our bodies don't respond as they once did. This struggle with weight can affect not just our physical well-being but our mental and emotional health as well, leading to a cycle of self-doubt and frustration.

Intermittent fasting presents a promising solution to this persistent issue, offering a sustainable approach to weight management that aligns with the body's natural rhythms. By creating a caloric deficit without deprivation, fasting allows for more effective weight control. It enables the body to enter a state of fat burning, where stored fat becomes the primary fuel source. This process promotes fat loss while preserving lean muscle mass, essential for maintaining overall health as we age. Unlike traditional dieting, which often focuses on calorie restriction, fasting relies on timing to achieve its effects. This approach reduces the stress associated with constant calorie counting, allowing you to enjoy food without guilt. The emphasis shifts from restriction to balance, supporting a healthier relationship with food and eating patterns.

The stories of women who have successfully managed their weight through fasting testify to its efficacy. Take, for instance, the narrative of Lisa, who found herself losing inches from her waist after months of feeling stuck. She embraced fasting as part of her daily routine and noticed a change in her waistline and overall body composition. The weight she lost was predominantly fat, leading to a more toned and healthier appearance. Similarly, Kellie shared how fasting improved her body composition, allowing her to shed fat while maintaining muscle. These successes highlight the potential of fasting to transform not just weight but overall health and self-esteem.

Sustaining weight loss through fasting requires consistency, mindfulness, and a balanced approach to healthy living. Staying consistent with fasting helps reinforce new habits and supports your body's natural ability to regulate weight effectively. Mindful eating complements this process by encouraging awareness of hunger cues and fostering healthier food choices. By tuning into what and when you eat, you create a sustainable foundation for long-term success. Regular physical activity further enhances the benefits of fasting by boosting metabolism and preserving muscle health. Whether it's a brisk walk, a dance class, or strength training, staying active keeps your body

strong and resilient. Together, these strategies create a harmonious approach to maintaining weight loss, empowering you to enjoy lasting health and vitality.

IMPROVING SLEEP AND REDUCING STRESS WITH FASTING

Sleep disruptions and stress are two interconnected challenges of menopause, creating a cycle where each one exacerbates the other. Our dietary habits often play a significant role in this cycle. The foods we consume can influence the production of cortisol, the stress hormone, directly impacting our sleep patterns. Elevated cortisol levels, often due to stress or poor dietary choices, can make it difficult to fall asleep or stay asleep through the night. Additionally, consuming heavy meals before bed can disrupt sleep, as our bodies focus energy on digestion rather than rest, leading to fitful nights and groggy mornings.

Intermittent fasting offers a refreshing approach to breaking this cycle, promoting better sleep and reducing stress. By regulating circadian rhythms, fasting helps align our sleep-wake cycles with natural light patterns, encouraging more restful sleep. This alignment reduces nighttime awakenings, allowing the body to experience deeper, more restorative sleep. Moreover, fasting supports cortisol regulation, helping to level out those peaks and troughs that can leave us feeling frazzled and worn out. Many women, myself included, have found that incorporating fasting into our routines has led to a noticeable improvement in sleep quality. The quiet hours of fasting provide a respite from the constant demands of digestion, allowing the body to focus on healing and restoration.

Take Ellen's experience, for example—she struggled with persistent insomnia and anxiety, feeling trapped in an exhausting cycle. But after adopting intermittent fasting, she noticed a shift. Her sleep became more consistent, and her nighttime anxiety gradually eased. The structure of her fasting routine helped her body establish a natural rhythm, leading to more restful nights and calmer days. Similarly, Kimberly shared how fasting alleviated her nighttime anxiety, allowing her to fall asleep more easily. These stories highlight a common theme: fasting nourishes the body and soothes the mind, fostering a sense of balance that promotes restful sleep and overall well-being.

To optimize sleep and manage stress effectively, consider incorporating lifestyle changes that complement your fasting practice. Establishing a bedtime routine can signal to your body that it's time to wind down, helping you transition smoothly from the busyness of the day to the tranquility of the night. This routine might include gentle activities like reading, taking a warm bath, or practicing relaxation techniques. Mindfulness practices, such as meditation or deep breathing exercises, can further support stress reduction, encouraging a state of calm that facilitates restful sleep. Regular exercise, such as walking or yoga, provides another layer of support, promoting physical health and emotional well-being. These activities help regulate the body's natural rhythms, enhancing the benefits of fasting and creating a foundation for improved sleep.

Reducing caffeine and alcohol intake can also significantly impact sleep quality. Both substances can interfere with the body's ability to relax and enter deep sleep, leading to fragmented rest and a lack of rejuvenation. Limiting these stimulants, particularly in the hours leading up to bedtime, creates a more serene internal environment that welcomes sleep rather than resists it. Through these mindful adjustments, you can transform not only your relationship with sleep but also your overall experience of stress, finding balance and peace in the rhythm of daily life.

SUPPORTING HEART HEALTH THROUGH FASTING

Heart health becomes a focal point of our well-being as we age, especially for women over 50. The risk of cardiovascular issues like hypertension and elevated cholesterol levels tends to rise, creating a landscape where vigilance and proactive care are crucial. Hypertension, or high blood pressure, can silently damage blood vessels, leading to serious conditions such as heart disease and stroke. Elevated cholesterol, particularly LDL cholesterol, contributes to plaque buildup in arteries, increasing the risk of heart attacks. These concerns often feel like an inevitable part of aging, casting a shadow over our health aspirations. However, understanding these risks is the first step toward managing them effectively, and intermittent fasting offers a promising avenue for support.

Intermittent fasting can significantly benefit heart health by positively impacting cardiovascular markers. One of the most notable benefits is the improvement in lipid profiles. Fasting encourages the body to shift from glucose to fat as a primary energy source, leading to lower LDL cholesterol and triglyceride levels. This shift helps reduce arterial plaque buildup, promoting healthier blood vessels. Furthermore, fasting has been shown to reduce blood pressure levels, offering a natural method to manage hypertension. This reduction stems from decreased insulin levels, leading to less sodium retention and improved kidney function. These changes create a heart-friendly environment, supporting cardiovascular health holistically and sustainably.

The scientific community has increasingly recognized the cardiovascular benefits of fasting, with numerous studies highlighting its positive effects. Research has demonstrated that fasting can significantly reduce cholesterol levels, supporting heart health in a way that aligns with the body's natural processes (Harvard Health, 2024). Experts in cardiology often endorse fasting as a viable strategy for reducing cardiovascular risk, emphasizing its role in improving blood pressure and lipid profiles. These insights provide a foundation of credibility and reassurance, underscoring fasting as a method backed by evidence and expert validation. This support can be empowering and encouraging for women navigating the complexities of heart health.

Consider integrating more heart-healthy habits into your daily routine to support cardiovascular health further while fasting. Cardiovascular exercise, such as brisk walking, cycling, or swimming, strengthens the heart and improves circulation. Regular physical activity is a cornerstone of cardiovascular health, supporting weight management and reducing stress. Reducing sodium intake is another important consideration, as excess sodium can elevate blood pressure. Focus on fresh, whole foods rather than processed options, which often contain hidden salts. A plant-focused diet, rich in fruits, vegetables, whole grains, and healthy fats, provides the nutrients necessary for heart health, supporting overall well-being.

Engaging in mindfulness practices can also significantly reduce stress, a known risk factor for heart disease. Techniques like meditation, deep breathing, or yoga promote relaxation and help manage stress levels, creating a calming effect that benefits the heart. By integrating these practices into your daily routine, you create a comprehensive approach to heart health that complements the benefits of fasting. This holistic perspective recognizes the interconnectedness of body and mind, offering a pathway to health that is both nurturing and empowering.

As we conclude this exploration of how fasting supports heart health, it's clear that this practice offers more than just a temporary fix. It aligns with the body's natural rhythms, promoting health in a way that feels intuitive and sustainable. The benefits of fasting extend beyond the physical, touching on the mental and emotional aspects of well-being. By embracing fasting as part of a heart-healthy lifestyle, you create a foundation for health that supports you through the years, empowering you to live with vitality and confidence. With this understanding, we move forward, ready to embrace the next chapter in our journey toward comprehensive well-being.

SHARE YOUR THOUGHTS: YOUR REVIEW MATTERS
EMBRACE THE GIFT OF GIVING

"The best way to find yourself is to lose yourself in the service of others."

— MAHATMA GANDHI

Reflecting on my own path, I understand the challenges and triumphs of embracing a new lifestyle, especially for women over 50. Your experiences with "The Essentials of Intermittent Fasting for Women 50 & Beyond" are invaluable. By sharing your review, you can inspire and guide others who are curious yet hesitant.

Many readers rely on reviews to make informed choices. Your insights can:

- Empower another woman to regain her vitality.
- Support a small business dedicated to women's health.
- Encourage an entrepreneur striving to make a difference.
- Provide meaningful work for those passionate about wellness.
- Help a reader transform her life and well-being.

Taking a moment to leave a review costs nothing but can profoundly impact someone else's journey. To share your thoughts, simply scan the QR code below and let your voice be heard:

Together, we can create a ripple effect of positive change.

Thank you for being a part of this community.

With heartfelt gratitude,

Jessica Christine

5
MENTAL CLARITY AND EMOTIONAL WELL-BEING

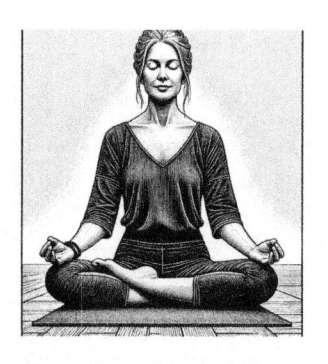

Have you ever walked into a room and completely forgotten why you were there? Or you've caught yourself rereading the same sentence multiple times, unable to focus. These moments of mental fog are all too familiar for many women over 50 and are not just frustrating but often disheartening. In these times, exploring intermittent fasting can offer a path back to clarity and focus. While the transformation doesn't happen overnight, with time, you may notice your mind becoming sharper, your concentration improving, and a renewed sense of mental energy emerging.

Intermittent fasting has been shown to enhance cognitive functions, offering a beacon of hope for those of us seeking to clear the fog. One key player in this process is the increased production of brain-derived neurotrophic factor (BDNF), a protein that supports the growth and survival of neurons. BDNF acts as a fertilizer for the brain, encouraging the development of new connections and enhancing synaptic plasticity, which is essential for learning and memory (Prevention, 2024). This means that fasting helps maintain the neurons you have and encourages the formation of new ones, contributing to improved memory retention. It's akin to giving your brain a tune-up, fine-tuning the processes that keep your mind agile and sharp.

Beyond BDNF, fasting promotes autophagy, the body's natural process of cleaning out damaged cells, including those in the brain. This cellular clean-up supports brain health by reducing inflammation and removing cellular debris that can contribute to cognitive decline. The reduction in brain fog many women experience is often attributed to this process, as it allows the brain to function more efficiently. Moreover, fasting helps stabilize blood sugar levels, preventing spikes and crashes that disrupt focus and attention. With a more stable energy supply, your brain can maintain concentration for extended periods, allowing you to engage fully in tasks without the constant distraction of hunger or fatigue.

Fasting offers another powerful benefit through the production of ketones—an alternative fuel source for the brain. Ketones provide a steady, efficient energy supply, enhancing mitochondrial function and optimizing brain performance. This improved energy efficiency can lead to sharper mental clarity, making once-daunting tasks more manageable. Many women describe experiencing a renewed sense of focus, as if a mental fog has lifted, allowing their thoughts to feel clearer and more precise than they have in years.

Take, for instance, the story of Diane, a woman who improved her work performance after integrating intermittent fasting into her routine. As a marketing executive, Diane was accustomed to multitasking and managing complex projects, but brain fog had started to hinder her efficiency. After a few months of fasting, she noticed a significant improvement in her ability to concentrate and precisely complete tasks. Her colleagues even commented on her newfound focus and creativity, a testament to the cognitive benefits she experienced.

To maximize the cognitive benefits of fasting, consider incorporating omega-3-rich foods into your diet. Foods like hemp seeds, flaxseeds, walnuts, soybeans, spinach, and brussel sprouts provide essential fatty acids that support brain health and cognitive function. Regular mental exercises, like puzzles, reading, or learning a new skill, can also help keep your mind sharp. Engaging in mindfulness practices, such as meditation or yoga, further supports mental clarity by reducing stress and promoting relaxation. By quieting the mind, these practices enhance your ability to focus and think clearly. Lastly, ensure you get adequate sleep, as rest is essential for memory consolidation and cognitive performance.

Incorporating these practices into your fasting lifestyle creates a holistic approach to mental clarity, allowing you to enjoy the full benefits of fasting. As you explore these strategies, remember that mental clarity is not just about sharper thinking—it's about feeling more connected to yourself and the world around you. Embrace this opportunity to nurture your mind and reclaim the mental agility that enhances every aspect of life.

EMOTIONAL BALANCE: FASTING AS A TOOL FOR STABILITY

The emotional ups and downs that come with life after 50 can feel like standing at the edge of a storm—unpredictable and overwhelming, never quite knowing when the winds will settle. Many of us have experienced this emotional whirlwind, and through countless conversations and shared stories, I've discovered how intermittent fasting can bring a sense of balance amidst the chaos. At its core, fasting helps regulate mood-related hormones, fostering a steadier emotional foundation and offering a much-needed sense of calm and clarity. By influencing hormones such as serotonin and dopamine, fasting can reduce anxiety and depressive symptoms, offering a more tranquil internal landscape. This modulation helps to clear the emotional clutter, paving the way for a more peaceful and balanced existence.

Fasting also plays a pivotal role in stress management, acting as a natural buffer against the pressures of daily life. One of the mechanisms behind this is its effect on cortisol, the hormone often dubbed the "stress hormone." Fasting lowers cortisol levels, which can lead to a reduction in stress and anxiety. With decreased inflammation markers, fasting promotes a sense of calm and control, allowing you to face challenges with a steadier hand. It's like finding a quiet center in a world full of noise where you can breathe deeply and exhale stress. This physiological response reduces stress and fosters an environment where emotional stability can flourish.

Ivy is a woman who struggled with constant mood swings that left her feeling emotionally drained. Before embracing intermittent fasting, she often felt like she was on an unpredictable seesaw, swinging between highs and lows that disrupted her daily life. But after several months of fasting, she noticed a profound shift—her mood swings became less intense and far less frequent. With a newfound sense of emotional stability, Ivy felt more at peace, able to fully engage in her relationships and daily activities without the constant emotional turbulence. Her story is a powerful reminder of how fasting can help restore balance, offering a more harmonious and fulfilling way of living.

For those seeking to maintain emotional balance, there are several strategies you can incorporate into your everyday routine. One such practice is gratitude journaling, a simple yet profound way to focus on the positive aspects of life. By writing down what you're grateful for each day, you can shift your perspective and cultivate a more positive outlook. This practice isn't about ignoring challenges but acknowledging the good that exists alongside them. Engaging in regular physical activity is another key strategy. Exercise releases endorphins, the body's natural mood enhancers, and provides a healthy outlet for stress. Whether it's a brisk walk in the park or a gentle yoga session, finding movement that you enjoy can significantly improve your mood and emotional resilience.

Incorporating yoga and meditation into your routine can further support emotional stability. These practices encourage mindfulness, helping you become more aware of your thoughts and emotions without judgment. They offer a space to breathe deeply and release tension, creating a sanctuary of calm amidst life's demands. With its combination of movement and breathwork, yoga can be particularly effective in reducing stress and fostering a sense of connection with the body. Conversely, meditation provides a quiet space for reflection, allowing you to observe your thoughts and emotions with a sense of detachment. Together, these practices can form a cornerstone of emotional well-being, supporting you as you navigate the complexities of life with grace and ease.

MINDFUL EATING: ENHANCING YOUR FASTING EXPERIENCE

Visualize sitting at your dining table, the outside world's noise fading away as you bring your focus inward. This is the essence of mindful eating—a practice that invites you to engage fully with each meal, heightening your awareness and appreciation of the food before you. Mindful eating complements intermittent fasting perfectly, amplifying the benefits of both practices. Concentrating on the sensory experience of eating, you cultivate a deeper connection with your body and its needs. Ask yourself, "Is this food nourishing my body?" This question prompts you to choose foods that support your health and wellness, guiding you toward more nutritious options. Avoiding distractions during meals becomes an act of self-care, allowing you to savor each bite without the pull of daily stressors.

The benefits of mindful eating are profound, particularly in the realms of digestion and satiety. When you slow down and truly engage with your meal, digestion improves. A slower eating pace gives your body time to break down food, reducing discomfort and bloating properly. Recognizing hunger and fullness cues becomes second nature, helping you avoid overeating and promoting a healthy relationship with food. This awareness increases satisfaction with smaller portions as you learn to trust your body's signals and respond accordingly. Mindful eating turns meals into a meditative experience, where each bite is an opportunity to deepen your understanding of nourishment and satiety.

Transform your meals into a moment of mindfulness by creating a calm, distraction-free space—turn off the TV, put your phone aside, and allow yourself to be fully present. Before taking your first bite, pause for a deep breath, grounding yourself in the experience. As you eat, slow down and savor each mouthful—notice the textures, flavors, and aromas unfolding with every bite. Engage all your senses, appreciating the vibrant colors on your plate and the intricate layers of taste. Tune into your body's signals, recognizing when you feel satisfied and permitting yourself to stop eating without guilt or obligation. By embracing this intentional approach, every meal becomes an opportunity to nourish your body and mind.

Reflect on Laura's narrative. Laura found that mindful eating helped her reduce overeating, a habit she had struggled with for years. By focusing on the sensory aspects of her meals, Laura became more attuned to her body's signals, recognizing when she was truly hungry and when she had eaten enough. This awareness allowed her to break free from the cycle of emotional eating, replacing it with a deliberate and joyful approach to nourishment. Laura's journey highlights the transformative potential of mindful eating, offering a path to greater self-awareness and healthier eating habits.

As you explore mindful eating, remember that it is a practice, not a destination. Each meal is an opportunity to reconnect with your body and honor its needs. By integrating mindfulness into your fasting routine, you can enhance the benefits of both practices, creating a harmonious relationship with food that supports your well-being. This balance between mindfulness and fasting offers a holistic approach to health, one that nourishes both body and soul. Embrace this practice with an open heart, allowing it to guide you toward a deeper understanding of yourself and your relationship with food.

BUILDING RESILIENCE: COPING WITH AGING CHALLENGES

We often admire resilience in others but may overlook it in ourselves. That inner strength allows you to face adversity, adapt, and emerge stronger. Intermittent fasting can play a surprising role in fostering this resilience, particularly as we age. By strengthening mental fortitude, fasting helps you build a robust internal framework that supports emotional and psychological well-being. This fortitude reduces impulsive behaviors, allowing you to respond to life's challenges with thoughtfulness rather than reactiveness. Fasting encourages an adaptive stress response, teaching your body and mind to handle stress more effectively. This adaptability is crucial, as it helps you maintain stability amidst the inevitable changes and challenges of aging.

The benefits of resilience extend far beyond the ability to weather storms; they enrich every aspect of life. Developing resilience can enhance your quality of life, particularly as you face aging transitions. It provides the ability to handle these changes with composure, transforming potential stressors into opportunities for growth. Imagine confidently navigating retirement, embracing the freedom and possibilities it presents rather than fearing the loss of routine. Resilience also helps build self-esteem, empowering you to recognize your worth and capabilities. As you gain confidence, stress and worry diminish, replaced by a positive outlook that colors your interactions and decisions. This positivity is not a denial of difficulty but a recognition of your strength and potential to overcome it.

Consider the story of Ellen, a woman who, through fasting, discovered a newfound resilience that carried her through retirement. Initially apprehensive about leaving the workforce, Ellen feared losing her identity and purpose. Yet, fasting helped her build the mental fortitude she needed to embrace this new chapter with enthusiasm. Ellen began volunteering at a local charity, channeling her skills and energy into meaningful work. This shift filled her days with purpose and reinforced her resilience, proving that she could adapt and thrive in any circumstance. Another testimonial comes from Monika, who faced significant health challenges. Fasting became a tool for her to regain control over her health, strengthening her resolve and helping her overcome obstacles with determination. These stories are about survival and thriving, highlighting how fasting can support a resilient mindset.

Building resilience starts with setting achievable goals that provide direction and purpose. By breaking more considerable challenges into manageable steps, goals create a clear path forward, keeping you focused and motivated. Whether you commit to a daily walk, learn a new skill, or explore a creative project, these small, intentional steps can lead to meaningful progress.

Equally important is the practice of self-reflection. Processing your experiences and emotions allows you to learn, adapt, and make choices that align with your values. By recognizing patterns and understanding yourself more deeply, you empower yourself to navigate challenges more clearly and confidently.

As you integrate these strategies into your life, remember that resilience is not a fixed trait but a dynamic process. It's about cultivating an inner reservoir of strength that you can draw upon when needed. By embracing fasting as a tool for resilience, you empower yourself to face aging challenges with courage and grace.

FINDING JOY IN FASTING: CULTIVATING A POSITIVE MINDSET

Embracing intermittent fasting can be transformative, but the true magic happens when you cultivate a positive mindset. Instead of seeing fasting as a challenge to endure, reframe it as an opportunity to nourish and empower your body. When you approach fasting with gratitude, the experience shifts from restriction to growth and renewal.

Take a moment to appreciate what your body is capable of—each day is a chance to celebrate small victories, whether feeling more energized, experiencing greater mental clarity, or simply moving through your day with a lighter step. By focusing on these positive changes, fasting becomes a practice you genuinely look forward to, nurturing your body and sense of fulfillment.

Viewing fasting as a path of discovery rather than a restrictive task opens the door to personal growth. You begin to uncover new strengths and capabilities, realizing you're capable of more than you ever imagined. Each fasting day becomes a chance to learn about yourself and to understand your body's signals and needs more deeply. It's a journey of self-exploration, where you discover the resilience and determination within you. Celebrating small victories along the way reinforces this growth. Whether completing your first week of fasting or noticing an improvement in your mood, these achievements build confidence and motivation.

Consider the story of Jenna, who found unexpected empowerment through fasting. Initially skeptical, Jenna approached fasting with caution, unsure of what to expect. Yet, as the weeks passed, she discovered a joy she hadn't anticipated. Fasting became a source of empowerment, strengthening her sense of self. She felt more in tune with her body's rhythms and embraced the changes she observed. Jenna's experience highlights the joy that can be found in fasting, a joy that stems from self-awareness and growth.

To cultivate joy and positivity in your fasting practice, start gradually. Allow yourself the grace to adjust to this new lifestyle at your own pace. There's no rush, and each step forward is a success in itself. Practicing daily affirmations further supports a positive mindset. Simple statements like "I am strong" or "I am capable" reinforce your belief in yourself and your ability to thrive. Listening to your body's signals is another key element. Pay attention to what your body needs, whether rest, hydration, or nourishment, and respond with kindness and care. This attentiveness fosters a nurturing relationship with your body, enhancing your fasting experience.

Joining a supportive community can make your fasting journey even more rewarding. Connecting with others who share similar goals and experiences provides encouragement, camaraderie, and a sense of belonging, reminding you that you're not alone. Engaging in shared conversations, exchanging stories, and celebrating challenges and victories can be incredibly motivating, offering fresh insights and inspiration. This collective support strengthens your commitment, helps you stay on track, and nurtures a positive mindset, especially during the more challenging moments.

MENTAL CLARITY AND EMOTIONAL WELL-BEING

As you cultivate joy in fasting, remember that it's about the journey, not the destination. It's about embracing the process, finding happiness in the present moment, and celebrating the growth of each step forward. By nurturing a positive mindset, you transform fasting into a fulfilling and joyful experience that enriches your life in countless ways.

With the foundation of mental clarity and emotional well-being firmly in place, Chapter 6 introduces the concepts of overcoming obstacles and staying motivated.

6

OVERCOMING OBSTACLES AND STAYING MOTIVATED

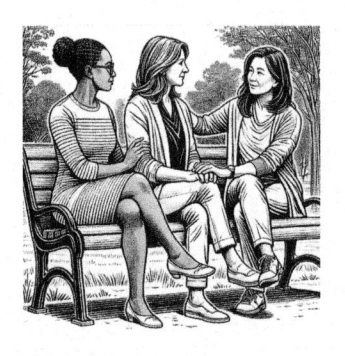

At some point in your fasting journey, you may encounter a plateau—a moment where progress seems to stall despite your consistency and discipline. It can feel like hitting a brick wall, with the scale refusing to budge no matter how dedicated you are. In these moments of frustration, remember that you're not alone. Many women face this same challenge, and it's a natural part of the process. Plateaus occur as the body adapts to change, and understanding why they happen is the first step toward breaking through and continuing your progress.

Fasting plateaus often result from the body's remarkable ability to adapt to new routines and conserve energy. Initially, when you begin fasting, your body responds by burning stored fat for fuel, leading to weight loss. However, over time, your metabolism may slow down in response to decreased caloric intake, a phenomenon known as adaptive thermogenesis. This slowdown can make further progress challenging, as it reduces the number of calories burned at rest. Hormonal changes, particularly decreases in leptin, a hormone that regulates hunger and metabolism, can also play a role. These physiological adaptations can make it feel like your progress has come to a screeching halt, even if you're diligently following your fasting plan (Prevention, 2024).

To break through this stagnation, consider shaking up your routine. Altering your fasting schedule can introduce a new challenge for your body, preventing it from becoming too comfortable with a set pattern. If you've been following a 16:8 schedule, try switching to a slightly different routine, such as a 5:2 plan, where you usually eat for five days and fast for two. This variation can kickstart your metabolism and reignite weight loss. Intermittent calorie cycling is another effective strategy. You can prevent your metabolism from slowing down by varying your caloric intake on different days. This means having days when you consume more calories, balanced with lower-calorie days. It's like giving your metabolism a wake-up call, reminding it to stay active and engaged.

Physical activity is a powerful tool for breaking through plateaus. Increasing the intensity or frequency of your workouts can help counteract a slowing metabolism while incorporating resistance training, which builds muscle—boosting calorie burn even at rest. Equally important is prioritizing quality sleep. Lack of rest disrupts hunger and metabolism-regulating hormones, making it harder to push past a plateau. Managing stress is another key factor, as elevated cortisol levels can encourage fat storage, especially around the abdomen. Nutrition also plays a vital role. A balanced, plant-focused diet rich in nutrients supports your body's needs and enhances your fasting efforts. Fiber- and protein-rich foods promote satiety, helping you stay full longer, curb overeating, and maintain steady energy levels. Combining these strategies creates a well-rounded approach to overcoming plateaus and continuing your progress.

Patience and persistence are vital during these times. It's easy to feel discouraged when progress stalls, but remember that your body is adjusting and recalibrating. Understanding the body's adaptive mechanisms can alleviate some of the frustration. This knowledge empowers you to remain committed, recognizing that plateaus are temporary and surmountable. Reassess your goals and remind yourself of the progress you've already made. Each step forward is a testament to your dedication and resilience.

Consider the story of Rachel, a woman stuck in a plateau after months of steady weight loss. She tweaked her fasting schedule, incorporating one longer fast each week. This small change made a significant difference. Within weeks, Rachel began to notice her clothes fitting more loosely, and the scale started moving again. Her renewed progress was a powerful reminder of the importance of flexibility and adaptation in her fasting journey. Rachel's experience illustrates that overcoming plateaus is about finding what works for you, staying open to change, and trusting in the process.

REFLECTION EXERCISE: NAVIGATING YOUR PLATEAU

Pause to assess your current fasting routine. How could you introduce some variation to present a new challenge to your body? Note any potential adjustments you are open to exploring, such as modifying your fasting schedule, tweaking your nutritional intake, or amplifying your exercise regimen. Record your advancements and emotional journey throughout this process. Use this reflective exercise to keep your determination sharp and your spirit engaged.

SOCIAL SITUATIONS: NAVIGATING DINING OUT AND EVENTS

Picture this: you're at a lively dinner party, surrounded by laughter and the clinking of glasses. The aroma of rich foods fills the air, tempting your senses. Yet beneath the surface, there's a subtle tension. The pressure to conform to group dining habits is palpable. Friends insist, "Just have a bite; it won't hurt." It's a familiar scenario for many of us embracing intermittent fasting. Social settings often challenge our resolve, testing the boundaries we've set for ourselves. Limited menu options can add to the stress. How do you stick to your fasting goals when everyone around you seems to be indulging? It's not just about the food; it's about navigating the cultural expectations to eat, share, and partake in the communal experience.

One of the most effective strategies for staying true to your fasting goals in social settings is to inform your family and friends about your fasting schedule ahead of time. Communication is key. Sharing your intentions creates a supportive environment where your choices are respected. This proactive approach sets clear expectations and opens up opportunities for dialogue. For instance, you might explain the benefits of fasting—how it's improved your energy, mood, and overall health. This can foster understanding and even spark interest among your loved ones. Choosing restaurants with fasting-friendly menu items can also ease the pressure. Look for places that offer various options, such as salads, grilled plant proteins, or vegetable-based dishes, allowing you to enjoy the meal without compromising your dietary choices.

In strategizing your social agenda, lean towards social engagements that don't revolve around meals. Opt for activities that foster connections without emphasizing eating, such as nature hikes, museum tours, or live music events. These alternatives allow for meaningful interactions minus the food-focused temptations. Consider bringing your preferred snacks in scenarios where food plays a central role. A compact container filled with nuts or fresh fruit can serve as a healthier choice, ensuring you stay true to your fasting commitments. Adaptability plays a key role here as well. Adjust your fasting window when anticipating significant social gatherings. Shifting your eating times slightly earlier or later can help you partake in special occasions without compromising your fasting progress.

Effective communication and planning are your allies in these situations. By explaining your fasting goals to loved ones, you enlist their support, making them partners in your journey rather than obstacles. Planning meals around social events can help maintain your routine, ensuring you're not caught off guard. This might mean having a light meal before going out so you're not ravenous and tempted to overindulge. The goal is to enjoy the social aspect without feeling deprived or pressured.

Consider the story of Helen, who attended a family reunion while maintaining her fasting schedule. Before the gathering, she informed her relatives about her commitment to fasting, explaining how it had transformed her health. Her family embraced her choices, ensuring plenty of options fit her needs. Helen brought a dish that she could enjoy, shared it with others, and demonstrated that fasting doesn't mean missing out on flavor or enjoyment. Her story underscores the critical role of preparation and clear communication in effectively managing the social aspects of fasting.

Navigating social situations while fasting is not about isolation but finding balance. It's about enjoying the company and the moment while honoring the commitments you've made to yourself. Remember that your health and well-being are worth the effort in these situations. You have the tools to maintain your goals without sacrificing your social life. With a bit of planning and a lot of communication, you can enjoy the best of both worlds, feeling confident and empowered in your choices.

STAYING MOTIVATED: TIPS FOR LONG-TERM ADHERENCE

Staying motivated with long-term fasting can sometimes feel like a battle against routine. The initial excitement of a new regimen may fade over time, leaving you feeling stuck in a cycle that no longer carries the same thrill. This frustration can be compounded by slow or invisible progress—when the scale doesn't budge or your reflection in the mirror looks unchanged, it's easy to wonder if the effort is even worth it. Beyond this, dehydration can quietly drain your energy, especially if you're not drinking enough water throughout the day, leading to fatigue that makes fasting more challenging. Over-restriction can take an even more significant toll, leaving you both physically depleted and mentally exhausted, making it tempting to abandon your goals. Recognizing these challenges is the first step toward overcoming them, allowing you to adjust your approach and reignite your motivation.

To keep your enthusiasm alive, focus on setting small, achievable milestones. These milestones act as stepping stones, guiding you along your path and providing a sense of accomplishment with each one you reach. Whether fasting for an extra hour or trying a new healthy recipe, each milestone is a victory in its own right. Celebrate these non-scale victories as they arise—fitting into an old pair of jeans, feeling more energetic, or simply enjoying a day without cravings. These moments remind you that progress isn't always about numbers; it's about how you feel and the subtle changes that occur along the way. Visualizing long-term health benefits can also serve as a powerful motivator. Picture yourself with increased vitality, participating in activities you love, and living with a newfound sense of ease. This vision can breathe new life into your passion and dedication.

Self-reflection and reevaluation are crucial to maintaining focus. Regularly take note of your successes and challenges. Writing can be a cathartic exercise, helping you process your experiences and gain insight into what works for you. Reflect on the highs and lows, and allow yourself to learn from each experience. These reflections remind you of your resilience and determination, offering a clearer perspective on your journey. Reevaluating your goals can also breathe new life into your routine, ensuring your objectives remain relevant and inspiring.

Motivational quotes and stories can provide the spark you need when your motivation wanes. Consider the words of a renowned health coach who once said, "Success is the sum of small efforts, repeated day in and day out." This quote emphasizes the power of consistency and the impact of incremental progress. Each day you commit to your fasting goals is a building block toward success. Take the story of Olivia, a woman who found herself losing interest in her fasting routine. Feeling uninspired, she began reading about others who had transformed their lives through fasting. These stories reignited her passion, and she found herself motivated once more. Olivia's experience highlights how connecting with the experiences of others can renew your enthusiasm and remind you of the possibilities that lie ahead.

As you journey forward, it's essential to understand that motivation naturally fluctuates, demanding continuous care and reinforcement. Concentrating on incremental achievements, picturing your objectives, and contemplating your advancements will help sustain the drive necessary for reaching your goals. Draw strength and encouragement from those who have embarked on similar paths, reassuring yourself of your inherent resilience, especially when motivation seems distant.

BUILDING A SUPPORT NETWORK: COMMUNITY AND CONNECTION

Visualize sitting in a cozy café, surrounded by a group of women who truly understand the highs and lows of fasting. The conversation flows effortlessly, filled with laughter, shared tips, and mutual encouragement. This is the power of community—the invisible backbone that sustains us when we feel like giving up. In the realm of fasting, a supportive network can make all the difference. Encouragement from like-minded individuals can lift your spirits on days when motivation wanes, reminding you that you're not alone in this pursuit. Engaging in exchanges facilitates personal development and progression, tapping into the collective wisdom of those who have walked the path before you. You can exchange meal ideas, discuss strategies for overcoming challenges, and celebrate each other's big and small victories.

Finding and building a support network begins with seeking out spaces where others share similar goals and interests. Online forums dedicated to fasting can be a treasure trove of advice and camaraderie. These platforms connect you with individuals from diverse backgrounds, all united by a common goal. You can participate in discussions, ask questions, and draw inspiration from the stories shared by others. If you prefer face-to-face interactions, consider joining local fasting support groups. These gatherings offer a sense of community and accountability, providing a space to connect with others in your area who are also exploring fasting. Being part of a virtual or in-person group allows you to share your journey with others who truly understand the unique challenges and triumphs that fasting brings.

Consider the story of Claire, who found strength and support in a fasting-focused online community. Initially hesitant to share her experiences, Claire soon discovered the encouragement and empathy she received from others was invaluable. She connected with women who had faced similar struggles, and their stories resonated with her deeply. Through this community, Claire found new recipes to try, learned strategies to overcome obstacles, and, most importantly, felt understood and supported. Her testimonial highlights the transformative power of community, illustrating how connection can sustain and inspire us in ways we never imagined.

Surrounding yourself with a community of supportive peers lays a strong foundation for encouragement and accountability, crucial elements in bolstering your intermittent fasting journey. These connections serve as a potent reminder that you are not navigating this path in isolation; your experiences and challenges are echoed in the lives of many others. They provide a nurturing environment for exploration, learning, and personal growth, reinforcing your dedication to fasting and enhancing your overall health. Engaging with online forums and local support groups allows you to cultivate relationships that become a source of strength and motivation, steering you through the fluctuations of your fasting experience. Embrace the strength of community to propel you towards your health and vitality goals.

PERSONALIZED SUCCESS STORIES: INSPIRATION FROM REAL WOMEN

Contemplate the profound connection you'd feel in a space surrounded by women, each sharing their distinct intermittent fasting journeys—stories of triumph, perseverance, and transformation that echo your experiences and aspirations. These stories are as diverse as the women themselves, coming from different backgrounds and starting points, each with their own goals and achievements. Take, for instance, Sandy, a retired teacher who had struggled with weight gain and fatigue for years. She began fasting, hoping to lose a few pounds, but found so much more. The clarity in her mind and the energy she regained were unexpected gifts that transformed her daily life. Fasting became more than a weight loss tool; it rejuvenated her zest for living, enabling her to engage in activities she thought were behind her.

Then, there's Jamila, who approached fasting from a different angle. With a family history of diabetes, her primary goal was to improve her health markers and lower her risk. Jamila's story is one of perseverance. She faced challenges, particularly around social gatherings where food was central. Yet, she learned to adapt, finding strength in her ability to manage her health consciously. Over time, she saw her blood sugar levels stabilize and her confidence grow. Her journey highlights the power of giving yourself grace, of knowing that each day is a step forward, even when it's not perfect.

These stories remind us of the importance of personal adaptation. No two paths are identical, and what works for one may not work for another. Fasting offers a framework, but the individual adjustments make it truly powerful. Whether altering fasting windows to fit a busy schedule or finding new recipes that make mealtimes enjoyable, the ability to adapt is crucial. It's about listening to your body and making choices that align with your lifestyle and goals.

Beyond physical changes, fasting has a profound impact on overall well-being. Women like Sandy and Jamila showcase how fasting can improve health markers such as cholesterol and blood pressure and enhance the quality of life. Fasting is about more than numbers on a scale; it's about feeling vibrant and alive, about waking up with energy and a sense of purpose. It can transform how you interact with the world, offering a renewed perspective on what's possible when prioritizing your health.

As you read these stories, consider the power of sharing your own. Documenting your fasting experience provides insight into your progress and serves as a source of inspiration for others. Platforms like online forums, social media, or journaling groups offer spaces to share your victories and challenges. Storytelling is a powerful tool for motivation. By sharing your journey, you contribute to a community of women who support each other, celebrate the highs, and navigate the lows together.

The lessons learned from these narratives are clear: perseverance is key, grace is essential, and adaptation is invaluable. Each woman's story illustrates that success is not a one-size-fits-all achievement but a personal triumph that reflects individual goals and circumstances. As you continue on your path, remember that your story holds the potential to inspire and uplift, to connect with others who may be walking a similar road. Embrace the opportunity to share, learn, and evolve, knowing your success is part of a larger tapestry of women's achievements.

REASSESSING GOALS: KEEPING YOUR JOURNEY FRESH

In any pursuit, especially as personal as fasting, regularly reassessing your goals is like checking the compass on a long hike. It ensures you're still heading in the direction that aligns with your evolving priorities and keeps the path interesting and challenging. Life is dynamic, and what you aimed for a few months ago might not resonate with where you are today. Your original goal was weight loss, but now you are more interested in boosting your energy levels or improving mental clarity. Keeping your goals relevant is critical to staying engaged and motivated. It's like refreshing the map to suit new terrains, ensuring that each step taken is purposeful and meaningful. This process isn't about discarding past aspirations but refining them to better fit the person you are becoming.

Setting meaningful and achievable goals starts with the SMART framework. This approach—Specific, Measurable, Achievable, Relevant, and Time-bound—provides a structured way to articulate your goal. For instance, instead of a broad goal like "improve health," consider something more specific, such as "increase daily energy levels by incorporating a 10-minute morning meditation routine within the next month." This clarity makes the goal tangible and provides a clear path forward. Leveraging technology can significantly enhance your fasting journey. Applications such as Body Fast, Fast Habit, and Window are equipped with functionalities that meticulously monitor your progress, offer timely reminders, and shed light on your fasting habits, seamlessly integrating with your daily routine to support and streamline your fasting experience. Regular progress reviews are essential, allowing you to celebrate successes and identify areas needing adjustment. They serve as checkpoints, affirming your journey and revealing how far you've come.

Embracing flexibility is fundamental to successful goal setting. The unpredictable nature of life means that rigid goals may become more of a hindrance than a help if they no longer align with your current situation. Allow yourself the grace to modify your goals as needed. This might mean extending a timeline to accommodate unexpected life events or shifting focus to a different area of health. Maintaining flexibility means viewing your goals as dynamic elements that grow and change alongside you. This flexibility minimizes stress and ensures that your fasting journey stays in harmony with your current life situation, ensuring that your endeavors continue to be gratifying and pertinent.

Reflect on Evelyn's journey, which began with an emphasis on shedding pounds. Over time, her priorities shifted as she discovered that enhancing her energy levels and sharpening her mental focus became paramount in her daily life. By reevaluating her objectives, Evelyn redirected her attention to incorporating nutrient-rich foods and embracing mindfulness practices. This pivot rejuvenated her commitment to fasting and infused her routine with a deeper sense of purpose, exemplifying the transformative potential of periodically reassessing one's goals. Over time, she realized that her energy levels and mental sharpness had become more important to her daily life than the number on the scale. Evelyn's story illustrates the power of goal reassessment and the benefits of aligning your efforts with what truly matters to you now.

As you continue your fasting path, remember that reassessing your goals is not a sign of indecision but of growth. It reflects your ability to listen to your body and mind, honor their needs, and make choices supporting your well-being. Each reassessment is an opportunity to realign with your vision and ensure that your efforts are directed toward what brings you joy and health. Your journey is unique, and so are your goals. Keep them fresh, and let them guide you toward a fulfilling and vibrant life. Looking ahead, we'll delve into how fasting can be seamlessly woven into holistic health practices, elevating your well-being and enriching your journey toward longevity.

7
INTEGRATING FASTING WITH HOLISTIC HEALTH PRACTICES

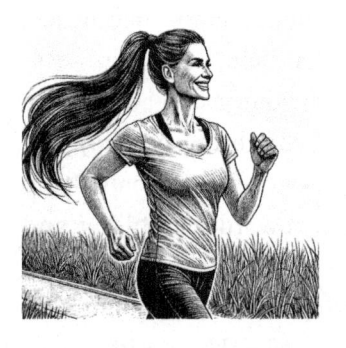

One afternoon after work, as I laced up my sneakers, I couldn't help but reflect on how much my relationship with exercise had transformed. What once felt like an obligation had become a gift—a way to honor my body through movement. Whether it was a walk outside or a session on the treadmill at the gym, I realized that this daily activity wasn't just beneficial—it was essential for my body and my spirit. Discovering how intermittent fasting and exercise practices could work together to enhance my well-being was a revelation. Exercise, it turns out, isn't just about burning calories or achieving a particular physique. It's about enhancing the benefits of fasting and vice versa, creating harmony that boosts physical and mental health. The most noticeable effect of integrating exercise with fasting is the boost in metabolic rate. When you exercise while fasting, your body is forced to use stored energy, primarily from fat, which enhances fat oxidation. This process not only aids in weight loss but also helps improve metabolic health by reducing visceral fat, which is linked to various health conditions. Beyond metabolism, exercise supports muscle growth, which is crucial as we age. By maintaining and building lean muscle mass, exercise helps counteract the natural muscle loss that occurs with age, preserving strength and vitality.

Timing your workouts can significantly impact the effectiveness of fasting. Morning workouts, executed before breaking your fast, can be particularly beneficial. Exercising on an empty stomach encourages your body to burn fat more efficiently, as glycogen stores are low. This method can enhance fat oxidation and improve endurance over time. However, listening to your body and adjusting according to your energy levels is essential. If you find morning workouts too taxing, consider low-intensity activities during fasting periods. Walking, stretching, or gentle yoga can maintain physical activity without overwhelming your system. On the other hand, high-intensity workouts should be reserved for eating windows when your energy and nutrient levels are replenished, allowing for optimal performance and recovery.

Listening to your body is paramount when integrating fasting and exercise. Each day may feel different, and it's crucial to recognize signs of fatigue or overexertion. Adjusting workout durations and intensities based on your daily condition can prevent burnout and injuries. Incorporating mindful exercises like yoga complements fasting by reducing stress and helps maintain flexibility and balance. This approach fosters a holistic view of health, focusing on what your body needs rather than rigid schedules.

REFLECTION EXERCISE: TUNING INTO YOUR BODY

Every day, dedicate a moment to reflecting on your physical and emotional state before and after exercising. Keep a journal to document your energy levels, emotional well-being, and bodily sensations or discomforts. This personal record will serve as a valuable tool, allowing you to tailor your exercise regimen more closely to your body's unique requirements.

Reflect on Karen's journey, a woman in her late fifties who integrated fasting with her fitness routine to surmount a lingering weight loss plateau. Initially, she encountered difficulties with energy levels during her exercise sessions, feeling fatigued more quickly than anticipated. By strategically adjusting her routine, Karen incorporated morning walks before breaking her fast and scheduled her strength training sessions for times within her eating window. This modification allowed her body to adapt gradually, improving her stamina and overall fitness. Over time, not only did Karen witness a breakthrough in her weight loss efforts, but she also experienced an enhancement in her endurance and a deeper appreciation for her body's capabilities. Her experience underscores the transformative effect of combining fasting with exercise, showcasing the potential for substantial physical and emotional growth.

Another inspiring example is Christine, who found that adding yoga to her fasting regimen helped her maintain balance and flexibility as she aged. Yoga became a form of moving meditation for her, providing physical benefits and a sense of peace and connection to her body. These testimonials underscore the transformative potential of combining fasting with exercise, empowering you to embrace a holistic approach to health that honors your body and nourishes your spirit.

MINDFULNESS AND MEDITATION: ENHANCING YOUR FASTING ROUTINE

Envision waking up to a quiet morning, where the only sound is your breath, steady and calm. This sense of peace can be the foundation of your day, especially when you pair mindfulness and meditation with fasting. These practices offer a sanctuary from the chaos of daily life, promoting mental clarity and emotional stability. Fasting, by its nature, can sometimes bring stress and anxiety as your body adjusts to new rhythms. Mindfulness helps diminish these feelings by anchoring you in the present moment, allowing you to observe your thoughts and emotions without judgment. Meditation can be a pause button, giving you space to breathe and regain composure. For many women, this combination becomes a powerful tool for navigating the challenges of fasting and life in general.

Mindfulness encourages you to tune into your body's true hunger and fullness cues, helping you break free from eating out of habit or emotion. This heightened awareness is especially valuable when fasting, as it allows you to understand your body's signals better. You can avoid unnecessary snacking and stay aligned with your fasting goals by recognizing genuine hunger. Beyond its impact on eating habits, mindfulness also sharpens focus and concentration, which can sometimes wane during fasting periods. Grounding yourself through meditation helps maintain mental clarity, keeping you present and productive throughout the day. This improved mental sharpness supports your fasting journey and enhances your overall well-being, making each day feel more intentional and fulfilling.

Integrating mindfulness into your fasting journey can begin effortlessly with mindful breathing exercises. Take a few moments each day to focus on your breath, feeling the rise and fall of your chest. This simple act can center your mind and body, reducing stress and promoting relaxation. Guided meditation sessions can be invaluable. They can help you explore deeper levels of relaxation and self-awareness as they lead you through visualization and breathing techniques. These guided moments provide clarity and peace, especially on days when fasting feels particularly daunting.

Mindfulness profoundly impacts eating habits, transforming how you experience food. It encourages you to savor flavors and textures, making meals a sensory delight rather than a routine task. This conscious approach to eating helps you recognize hunger and satiety signals, allowing you to nourish your body appropriately. By eating mindfully, you can enhance the fasting experience and ensure that meals are fulfilling and satisfying.

Tara is someone who found solace in meditation during her fasting periods. Struggling with the initial stress of fasting, she turned to mindfulness to find peace. Through daily meditation, Tara learned to embrace her hunger cues and found that her cravings diminished. Tara's fasting experience became richer and more rewarding, and she felt more connected to her body than ever before. Similarly, Cassandra discovered that mindfulness transformed her eating habits. By focusing on the flavors and textures of her meals, she ate less but enjoyed her food more. This shift supported her fasting goals and brought a deeper sense of contentment and gratitude to her life.

STRESS MANAGEMENT: TECHNIQUES TO COMPLEMENT FASTING

Incorporating stress management into your fasting regimen is akin to tuning an instrument, bringing harmony and balance to your overall well-being. Stress, as many of us know, can have a sneaky way of creeping into our lives, affecting everything from our mood to our health. When you manage stress effectively, you create an environment where fasting can shine, enhancing its benefits and promoting peace and resilience. One of the most immediate benefits of stress management is the reduction of cortisol levels. Cortisol, the stress hormone, can wreak havoc on your body, disrupting sleep, increasing blood sugar, and even contributing to weight gain. By actively managing stress, you help balance your hormonal state, supporting mental clarity and emotional stability. This balance fosters a greater sense of peace, allowing you to navigate life's challenges with more grace and less anxiety.

Incorporating practical stress management techniques into your fasting routine can enhance your overall well-being, creating a more holistic approach to health. As mentioned earlier, deep breathing exercises offer a simple yet powerful way to promote relaxation and balance. By focusing on your breath, you can calm the nervous system, reduce stress, and enhance your overall sense of well-being. Progressive muscle relaxation is another effective practice. It involves tensing and relaxing different muscle groups, promoting relaxation and releasing tension. Both techniques are easy to incorporate into your daily routine and can be particularly beneficial during fasting periods when you feel more vulnerable to stress. Gentle stretching or practicing yoga can also complement your fasting routine, offering physical and mental benefits. Yoga, in particular, reduces anxiety and improves flexibility and balance, enhancing your overall physical health. Drinking herbal teas and staying hydrated can further support your stress management efforts. Herbal teas like chamomile or lavender have calming properties, soothing both body and mind. Journaling, too, can provide emotional release, allowing you to process and express your feelings in a safe and private space.

Walking in nature is another powerful way to reduce stress hormone levels. Being in a natural setting can profoundly impact your mood and stress levels, offering a sense of peace and connection to the world around you. Light jogging, too, can effectively increase the production of endorphins, the body's natural feel-good chemicals. This boost in endorphins can elevate your mood and provide a sense of euphoria, reducing the impact of stress and promoting a positive outlook.

Jaime's experience is a compelling testament to the power of integrating stress management techniques with fasting. She discovered tranquility in her daily nature walks, which allowed her to decompress and rejuvenate. This simple yet effective strategy substantially decreased her stress levels, fostering a sense of ease and relaxation in her life. After a particularly stressful week, she decided to take a daily walk in her local park. The fresh air and serene environment provided a much-needed escape, allowing her to unwind and recharge. Over time, she noticed a significant reduction in her stress levels and felt more relaxed and at peace with her life.

SLEEP OPTIMIZATION: RESTFUL NIGHTS FOR BETTER DAYS

There's a profound connection between sleep and fasting that often goes unnoticed, especially in the hustle and bustle of our daily lives. Many women over 50 find themselves grappling with sleep disturbances, tossing and turning through the night, only to wake up feeling less than refreshed. Quality sleep is fundamental, not just for feeling well-rested, but for supporting the myriad benefits of fasting. Getting enough rest helps regulate key hormones, including insulin and cortisol, which play a vital role in overall health and are key players in managing blood sugar, appetite, and cravings. Achieving a balance in these hormones equips you with the resilience to navigate through the hunger associated with fasting periods and optimizes your body's energy utilization.

Additionally, adequate sleep significantly enhances mental well-being and vitality, crucial elements that empower you to meet the day with optimism and resilience. This aspect is particularly vital during fasting, influencing your perception and management of hunger. A well-rested mind possesses a stronger capacity for making healthful choices and adhering to fasting routines. Sleep facilitates bodily repair and rejuvenation, which are imperative when exercise is integrated, as it aids in muscle recovery and strengthening. Moreover, restorative sleep sharpens cognitive functions, improving focus and memory. This boost in mental acuity can transform your fasting journey from a challenging endeavor to an enriching experience of flourishing health, enhancing your ability to face the day with a positive mindset.

Adhering to a regular sleep routine is one highly effective method to enhance your sleep quality. This practice aids in synchronizing your body's internal clock, facilitating a smoother transition to sleep and wakefulness. Aim to go to bed and wake up at the same time each day, even on weekends. Creating a calming bedtime routine can also set the stage for restful sleep. Consider incorporating activities that relax the mind and body, such as reading a soothing book or taking a warm bath. Limiting screen time before bed is crucial, as the blue light emitted by phones and tablets can interfere with your ability to fall asleep. Instead, try practicing yoga or meditation before bedtime. These practices can calm the mind, reduce stress, and prepare your body for sleep.

Tracy, who had long struggled with insomnia, found that fasting, combined with a consistent sleep schedule, dramatically improved her sleep quality. By establishing a calming bedtime routine and practicing meditation, Tracy began experiencing deeper sleep and increased energy during the day. She felt more balanced and in control, her mind clear and focused. Similarly, Sophia, who frequently woke up during the night, discovered that limiting her screen time and incorporating yoga into her evening routine helped her achieve restful nights. She awoke feeling rejuvenated and ready to tackle the day's challenges with renewed vigor.

These stories illustrate the profound impact that optimizing sleep can have on fasting and overall health. They remind us that sometimes, the simplest changes can yield the most significant results. By prioritizing sleep, you enhance the benefits of fasting and improve your quality of life. Remember, your body does incredible work while you rest, regenerating and preparing for the day ahead. Embrace these sleep-enhancing practices to support your fasting efforts and overall well-being, nurturing a cycle of health that sustains and uplifts you.

GUT HEALTH: THE INTERPLAY WITH FASTING

Often referred to as the 'second brain,' the gut plays a powerful role in overall health, influencing far more than just digestion. A well-functioning gut optimizes nutrient absorption, ensuring your body gets the most from your foods—directly impacting energy levels and immune function. Beyond physical health, a balanced gut can also support mental well-being, helping to reduce stress and anxiety. It's incredible to consider that the trillions of bacteria in our intestines contribute to how our bodies operate and how we feel each day.

Fasting introduces a unique opportunity to support gut health by allowing the digestive system to rest and reset. During fasting, the digestive tract gets a much-needed break from processing food, which can alleviate symptoms of bloating and discomfort. This pause allows the body to utilize energy stored in fat cells, contributing to weight management and metabolic health. Additionally, fasting helps promote balance within the gut microbiome, the community of microbes that live in our intestines. A balanced microbiome supports digestive regularity, making it easier to maintain a comfortable and sustainable routine.

Consider incorporating fermented foods into your diet to support gut health during fasting. Fermented foods like yogurt, kimchi, and sauerkraut are rich in probiotics, beneficial bacteria that support gut balance. These foods can help replenish the gut microbiome, enhancing digestion and nutrient absorption. Staying hydrated is equally important, as water aids in the transport of nutrients and helps prevent constipation. Adding probiotics and prebiotics to your diet can further support gut health. Probiotics introduce beneficial bacteria, while prebiotics provide the necessary fuel for these bacteria to thrive. Foods high in fiber, such as fruits, vegetables, and whole grains, also play a key role. Fiber supports regular bowel movements and feeds the beneficial bacteria in the gut, promoting a healthy digestive environment. Conversely, minimizing processed foods and sugars can prevent gut imbalance and inflammation.

Rachel's experience is a powerful example. After years of struggling with digestive issues, she decided to try fasting. Within weeks, she noticed a significant improvement in her digestive comfort. Her bloating decreased, and she felt lighter and more energetic. By focusing on high-fiber foods and incorporating fermented options, Rachel supported her gut health and found a new sense of well-being. Similarly, Lois, who had dealt with irregularity for most of her life, started fasting and saw a remarkable change. Her digestion became more regular, and she no longer felt the discomfort that had been a constant companion. These stories highlight the powerful impact that fasting, paired with mindful dietary choices, can have on gut health.

EMBRACING LONGEVITY: FASTING FOR A LONGER, HEALTHIER LIFE

Fasting goes beyond simply losing weight or sharpening your mind—it's a powerful practice that supports overall well-being. It taps into the essence of longevity, supporting how long we live and how well we live those years. Fasting initiates a natural cleanup process within our cells by activating autophagy. Imagine your body as a bustling city; autophagy acts like a dedicated team of street sweepers, clearing away debris and leaving the pathways fresh and open. This cellular repair reduces the risk of chronic diseases, such as diabetes and heart disease, by eliminating damaged cells that can accumulate and cause inflammation. As we age, inflammation—often termed "inflammaging"—can accelerate aging and contribute to various health issues. Fasting helps reduce this oxidative stress, allowing your cells to breathe and function optimally.

The potential anti-aging benefits of fasting extend beyond cellular clean-up. By supporting healthy aging at the cellular level, fasting enhances physical vitality. It's like giving your cells a rejuvenating spa day, invigorating them to function as they did years ago. This profoundly affects energy levels and resilience, making everyday tasks less burdensome. Research suggests that fasting might slow aging processes, offering a glimpse into a future where age feels like a number, not a definition of our capabilities. Scientists have found that fasting impacts longevity by positively influencing metabolic pathways and stress resistance. These studies suggest that fasting could indeed extend the lifespan, but more importantly, it improves the quality of those years, promoting a life filled with vitality and vigor.

Experts in the field of cellular health, like Dr. Valter Longo, have highlighted the role of fasting in promoting a longer health span. They emphasize how fasting mimics certain aspects of calorie restriction, a well-known method for extending lifespan in various organisms. By implementing fasting, we can achieve similar benefits without the constant deprivation associated with traditional calorie restriction. The idea is not just to add years to our lives but to add life to our years. This focus on quality of life is what makes fasting such an appealing practice for those of us navigating the complexities of aging.

For many women, fasting has become a transformative experience, reinvigorating their sense of well-being and health. This practice invites us to embrace aging as a natural, positive process filled with opportunities for growth and renewal. As we step into this new chapter of life, fasting offers a gentle yet powerful way to support our bodies and minds, ensuring that we continue to thrive, regardless of age.

8
SCIENTIFIC INSIGHTS AND FUTURE PERSPECTIVES

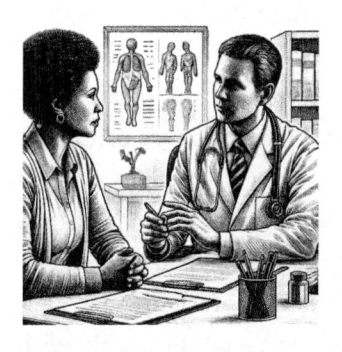

Experiencing firsthand how intermittent fasting enhanced many aspects of my life—and the lives of other women my age—sparked my curiosity and deepened my desire to understand the science behind this transformative practice. As women, we often seek evidence-based practices that resonate with our unique needs, especially as we age. It's not about following the latest trend but about making informed decisions supporting our health and well-being. This chapter delves into the scientific studies illuminating the benefits of intermittent fasting, offering a glimpse into the research supporting this powerful health approach.

Research has shown that intermittent fasting provides a wealth of benefits, particularly for women over 50. A comprehensive meta-analysis examining various fasting and metabolic health studies reveals that fasting can significantly improve metabolic markers. It enhances insulin sensitivity and promotes fat oxidation, making it a valuable tool for weight management. For many of us, these findings validate our experiences and provide a scientific foundation for our fasting practices. Longitudinal studies further support these claims, demonstrating that fasting not only aids in weight loss but also helps maintain it over time. These studies underscore fasting's potential as a sustainable method for achieving and maintaining a healthy weight, offering hope to those who have struggled with traditional diets.

When it comes to women over 50, specific studies have highlighted the unique benefits of intermittent fasting. Research focusing on post-menopausal women indicates that fasting can help balance hormones, reducing the frequency and severity of menopause-related symptoms. This is particularly significant, as hormonal changes during menopause can affect everything from mood to metabolism. Studies also indicate that fasting supports cognitive health, which is crucial as we age. By promoting cellular repair and reducing oxidative stress, fasting can enhance mental clarity and protect against age-related cognitive decline. These findings resonate deeply with many women, offering a scientific explanation for the cognitive improvements experienced during fasting.

In addition to these benefits, fasting has been linked to chronic disease prevention. Research suggests that intermittent fasting can reduce risk factors for cardiovascular disease, a leading cause of death among women. By improving cholesterol levels and lowering blood pressure, fasting supports heart health and reduces the risk of heart disease. Studies also indicate that fasting can lower markers of type 2 diabetes, a condition that often accompanies aging. By stabilizing blood sugar levels and enhancing insulin sensitivity, fasting offers a proactive approach to diabetes prevention. These findings are not just numbers on a page; they represent the potential for a healthier future, free from the burden of chronic disease.

REFLECTION SECTION: TRACKING YOUR FASTING JOURNEY

Record changes in your energy levels, mood, and overall physical health using a journal, notebook, or mobile app. Also, note any improvements in menopausal symptoms or mental clarity. This practice offers personal insights and helps you recognize patterns that align with broader scientific findings.

8.2 EXPERT OPINIONS: INSIGHTS FROM HEALTH PROFESSIONALS

Have you ever consulted an endocrinologist or watched interviews where they discuss how fasting can help support hormonal balance, especially during menopause—a stage often marked by challenging symptoms like hot flashes and mood swings? These experts emphasized that fasting helps regulate insulin and cortisol, providing stability to the hormonal fluctuations that many women face. This regulation not only aids in reducing those pesky symptoms but also contributes to an overall sense of well-being. The reassurance from these specialists that fasting is a safe practice for women over 50 is empowering. It offers a scientifically backed approach to managing health during a time when our bodies seem to have a mind of their own.

Conversations with plant-based nutritionists revealed fascinating recommendations for fasting meal plans. They highlighted the importance of incorporating nutrient-dense foods during eating windows, focusing on whole grains, legumes, fruits, and vegetables. These foods support fasting goals and promote heart health and longevity. The nutritionists I have learned from recommended including various colors and textures in meals to ensure a broad spectrum of nutrients. They also suggested mindful eating practices to enhance the fasting experience, such as savoring each bite and listening to the body's hunger cues. This holistic approach to nutrition during fasting aligns with the broader goal of fostering a healthy, balanced lifestyle.

Fasting's potential to extend health span and promote longevity is a topic that excites gerontologists. They highlighted how fasting influences cellular aging, slowing down the biological clock and enhancing the quality of life. By promoting autophagy, fasting aids in maintaining and repairing cells, which is essential for longevity. This cellular housekeeping can reduce the risk of age-related diseases, offering a path to a healthier, more vibrant life. Physicians further explained fasting's role in preventing chronic diseases. They discussed how fasting can lower the risk of heart disease and diabetes by improving metabolic health and reducing inflammation. These insights underscore fasting's potential as a preventative tool, providing hope for a future where age-related illnesses are less of a burden.

Professional endorsements of fasting's safety and efficacy come from various respected sources. Medical associations have issued statements confirming the benefits of fasting when practiced responsibly. These endorsements reassure that fasting is effective and safe, especially when guided by informed choices and professional advice. Health professionals, including dietitians and doctors, have spoken about fasting's ability to improve metabolic markers and enhance mental clarity. Their quotes often reflect a shared optimism

SCIENTIFIC INSIGHTS AND FUTURE PERSPECTIVES

about fasting's role in modern healthcare, encouraging its integration into wellness routines for women seeking a proactive approach to health.

Looking to the future, experts predict that fasting will become more integrated into healthcare practices. They foresee fasting protocols being adopted in medical settings, particularly for managing chronic conditions and supporting weight loss. As research continues to uncover fasting's benefits, it is expected to gain acceptance as a viable option for many health issues. This shift may lead to greater support from healthcare providers and broader access to resources that make fasting more accessible to everyone. The potential for fasting to revolutionize healthcare practices is exciting, offering a glimpse into a future where health and longevity are within reach for women everywhere.

8.3 FUTURE TRENDS: INNOVATIONS IN FASTING AND HEALTH

The world of fasting is continuously evolving, bringing forth innovations that make the practice more accessible and adaptable to individual needs. One of the most exciting trends is the development of tech-assisted fasting apps. These apps have transformed how we approach fasting, offering personalized guidance and tracking features that were once inconceivable. Imagine having a digital companion that tracks your fasting windows and offers valuable insights into your eating habits and progress. These apps often come equipped with features that allow you to log meals and track hydration and are now capable of monitoring fasting biomarkers, providing real-time feedback on how your body is responding to fasting. These devices can also monitor glucose levels, ketone production, and even heart rate variability, offering valuable insights into your metabolic health. For many women, especially those juggling busy schedules, these apps serve as a gentle guide, helping you stay on track without feeling overwhelmed.

Virtual fasting communities and support networks have also emerged, creating a sense of connection and accountability for those who prefer fasting in the company of others. These platforms allow users to share experiences, tips, and encouragement, fostering a community of like-minded individuals.

AI-driven health monitoring systems are another exciting development that is capable of offering personalized health recommendations based on your fasting data. These systems analyze patterns and trends, providing insights into nutrition, exercise, and stress management. Digital health platforms are being developed to offer a holistic approach to wellness, integrating fasting, exercise, and mindfulness practices into a comprehensive health plan. Biosensors for real-time metabolic monitoring are also on the horizon, promising to revolutionize how we understand and manage our health during fasting. These innovations represent a shift towards more informed and empowered fasting practices, enabling individuals to control their health proactively.

Another emerging trend is the rising interest in circadian rhythm fasting. This method aligns your eating schedule with your body's natural rhythms, promoting health by syncing with your internal clock. It emphasizes eating during daylight hours and fasting when it's dark, mimicking the natural ebb and flow of the day. The appeal of circadian rhythm fasting lies in its alignment with our biological processes, offering benefits like improved digestion and sleep, which are particularly appealing for women navigating the changes that come with aging. As more people become aware of the importance of circadian health, this method is gaining traction as a sustainable approach to fasting.

Advancements in personalized healthcare are also making waves in the fasting community. The use of genetic testing for tailored fasting plans is one such innovation. With a simple test, you can gain insights into your genetic predispositions, allowing for a fasting plan uniquely suited to your body's needs. This personalized approach considers factors like metabolism, hormonal balance, and even food sensitivities, ensuring that your fasting practice is safe and effective. For many women over 50, this level of customization offers peace of mind, knowing that their fasting plan is designed to support their individual health goals.

The intersection of fasting, technology, and personalized healthcare is paving the way for a new era of wellness. As these trends continue to evolve, they offer exciting possibilities for women over 50, providing tools and resources that make fasting more accessible and practical. Whether you're just starting your fasting journey or are a seasoned practitioner, these innovations offer new ways to engage with fasting, ensuring that it remains a dynamic and rewarding practice.

CREATING A LASTING LEGACY: FASTING AS A LIFESTYLE

In quiet moments of reflection, I often think about the future—not just my own but that of my family and future generations. What started as a simple health practice has evolved into a way of life, shaping my approach to wellness in a deeply meaningful way. Fasting isn't just a temporary solution; it's a sustainable practice that extends beyond the quick fixes of short-term diets. When seamlessly integrated into daily routines, fasting becomes as natural as brushing your teeth or taking a morning walk. Rather than a restriction, it becomes a source of balance, supporting long-term health and longevity while fitting harmoniously into everyday life.

The lifelong benefits of consistent fasting practices are profound. Over time, you may notice changes in your physical health and improvements in your mental and emotional well-being. Fasting has a way of bringing clarity and focus, helping you navigate the challenges of daily life with renewed energy and purpose. It fosters a deeper connection with your body, encouraging mindfulness and intentionality in every choice you make. This consistency builds a foundation for health that is resilient and adaptable, a legacy that can be passed down to future generations. As you embrace fasting as a lifestyle, you create a model of health that inspires those around you, demonstrating the power of small, consistent actions in achieving long-term wellness.

The impact of fasting on personal and familial health can create a ripple effect that extends far beyond your own life. When you prioritize your well-being, you set an example for your family, encouraging them to adopt healthier habits. It is not unusual for family members to develop a sense of curiosity, asking questions about the changes they observe in you. This curiosity can lead to conversations about health and wellness, opening the door to shared practices and mutual support. Fasting can become a family affair, a collective commitment to health that strengthens bonds and fosters a sense of community. This shared journey toward wellness can lead to transformative changes, with each member contributing to a healthier, more vibrant family dynamic.

SCIENTIFIC INSIGHTS AND FUTURE PERSPECTIVES

Take Jacqueline's story, for example—what started as a personal health practice soon evolved into a cherished family tradition. Her children, inspired by her dedication and the positive changes they saw, decided to join her in fasting. Together, they explored different fasting schedules and shared their experiences, learning from each other along the way. What started as a personal endeavor quickly blossomed into a multi-generational practice, with each family member finding their own path to health. Jacqueline's story speaks to the power of fasting to bring families together, creating a legacy of health that extends beyond the individual.

Education is essential for those looking to pass down the wisdom and benefits of fasting to younger family members. Hosting family fasting workshops can be a wonderful way to share knowledge and experiences, creating a space for open dialogue and learning. These workshops can be informal gatherings where family members discuss their fasting practices, share recipes, and support each other's goals. It's an opportunity to teach the principles of fasting in a supportive environment, fostering a sense of camaraderie and shared purpose. Creating legacy journals documenting fasting experiences is another way to preserve this knowledge. These journals can serve as a written record of personal insights, challenges, and triumphs, offering guidance and inspiration to future generations. By documenting your journey, you create a resource that family members can turn to for encouragement and advice, ensuring that the legacy of health and wellness continues to thrive.

EMPOWERMENT THROUGH KNOWLEDGE: CONTINUING YOUR JOURNEY

Knowledge is a powerful ally in your fasting practice, offering the tools and insights needed to navigate the complexities of health and wellness. As you engage with fasting, staying informed about the latest advancements in health research is crucial. Continuous learning helps you make informed decisions and adapt your fasting practices to suit your evolving needs. Consider enrolling in online health courses, which provide structured learning and access to expert insights on various aspects of health, including nutrition, exercise, and the science of fasting. These courses offer the opportunity to deepen your understanding and refine your approach, empowering you to take control of your health confidently.

Subscribing to health and wellness publications is another way to stay updated on the latest research and trends. These publications often feature articles by leading experts, offering evidence-based insights and practical advice. By keeping up with these resources, you can learn about new fasting methods, dietary recommendations, and lifestyle practices that support your health goals. Listening to podcasts focused on health is a convenient way to access information, especially if you're juggling a busy schedule. Many podcasts feature interviews with experts, providing a platform for diverse perspectives and inspiring stories that can motivate and guide you on your health journey.

To further support your learning, I've compiled a list of recommended books, articles, podcasts, and a valuable blog. These resources cover a range of topics related to fasting, nutrition, meal planning, and health, offering valuable insights and guidance. Engaging with these resources allows you to explore different aspects of fasting, from its impact on metabolic health to its role in supporting mental clarity and emotional well-being. By immersing yourself in this wealth of knowledge, you empower yourself to make informed choices and adapt your fasting practices to suit your individual needs better.

Additionally, active participation in health communities can enhance your fasting experience, providing support and encouragement along the way. Joining local health workshops or clubs allows you to connect with others who share your interests and goals. These gatherings provide a space for learning, sharing experiences, and building relationships with likeminded individuals. Participating in community wellness events can also inspire and motivate, offering exposure to new ideas and practices that can enrich your fasting journey.

Continuous learning is the cornerstone of an empowered fasting practice. By staying informed, engaging with health communities, and seeking inspiration from others, you cultivate a lifestyle that supports your health and well-being. This commitment to education and growth ensures that your fasting practice remains dynamic and adaptable, allowing you to navigate the challenges and opportunities that arise along the way. As you continue to explore the world of fasting, remember that knowledge is your ally, guiding you toward health and vitality.

CONCLUSION

As our journey together comes to a close, I want to take a moment to reflect on the transformative power of intermittent fasting. Throughout this book, we've explored the science behind fasting, the practical strategies for implementing it into your life, and the profound benefits it can offer for women over 50. We've discussed how fasting can support weight management, hormonal balance, mental clarity, and overall wellbeing. It's a powerful tool that enables us to take charge of our health and embrace a more intentional way of living.

The core concepts we've covered—from choosing the proper fasting schedule to nourishing your body with nutrient-dense foods—provide a foundation for success. By understanding the importance of personalizing your approach, listening to your body's needs, and staying committed to your goals, you can unlock the full potential of fasting. Remember, this journey is about progress, not perfection. Each small step you take towards better health is a victory worth celebrating.

CONCLUSION

As you reflect on the insights gained from this book, consider these key takeaways:

1. Fasting is a powerful tool for optimizing health, particularly for women over 50.
2. Choosing the proper fasting schedule that aligns with your lifestyle and goals is crucial.
3. Nourishing your body with whole, nutrient-dense foods during your eating windows is essential.
4. Addressing common challenges, such as hunger and social situations, is possible with the right strategies.
5. Fasting is not just about physical health; it can also enhance mental clarity and emotional well-being.

Now is the moment to move forward with intention. Establish achievable goals and devise a strategy tailored to your unique needs. Embrace the impact of gradual shifts—over time, these minor adjustments can lead to fundamental changes. Surround yourself with supportive peers who share your aspirations and are ready to offer motivation and guidance. Above all, practice self-compassion. This path is one of exploration and nurturing, not of self-critique.

As you begin this journey, remember that you are capable of remarkable things. Your body is resilient, and your mind is powerful. Each day, you'll become more in tune with your body's needs and more confident in making nourishing choices. Over time, fasting will feel effortless—a natural part of your lifestyle that empowers you to thrive and live your best life.

Envision a future where you wake up each morning feeling energized, clear-headed, and at peace with your body. A future where you have the vitality to pursue your passions, nurture

CONCLUSION

your relationships, and positively impact the world around you. That future is within reach, and fasting is a key that can help you unlock it.

So, my dear reader, I invite you to embrace this journey with an open heart and a curious mind. Trust in the process and trust in yourself. You have the power to transform your health and your life, one day at a time. Know that I am here, cheering you on every step of the way.

As we close this chapter together, I want to leave you with a final thought: Your health is your most incredible wealth. By prioritizing your well-being and committing to a lifestyle that supports your goals, you are investing in yourself and your future. You are worthy of vibrant health, boundless energy, and a life filled with joy and purpose.

So, take a deep breath, smile, and confidently step forward. Your journey to optimal health through intermittent fasting has only just begun, and I can't wait to see where it takes you.

With love and gratitude, Jessica Christine

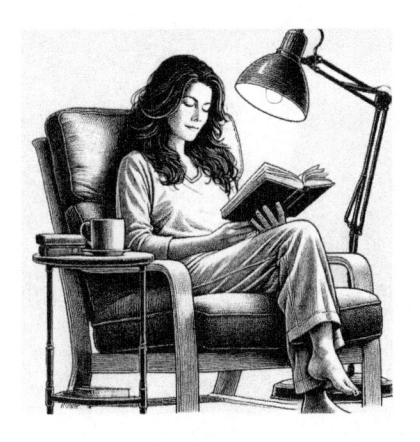

BOOK, WEBSITE & PODCAST RECOMMENDATIONS

- The China Study: The Most Comprehensive Study of Nutrition Ever Conducted and the Startling Implications for Diet, Weight Loss, and Long-term Health, by T. Colin Campbell
- Intermittent Fasting for Women Over 50 Mastery: A Proven Method for Weight Loss after Menopause, Anti-aging and Longevity (The Whole Foods Diet for Longevity Series), by Paul Griggs
- Exercise and Intermittent Fasting for Women Over 50 : Exercise and Intermittent Fasting for women after 50 with a plant-based diet meal plan (Hardcover), by Sarah Andersen
- https://www.pcrm.org/
- https://colleenpatrickgoudreau.com/food-for-thought-podcast/
- https://nutritionfacts.org/
- https://www.webmd.com/healthy-aging/what-to-know-about-intermittent-fasting-for-women-after-50
- https://telehealth.love.life/plant-based-doctors-qa-fasting-menopause-sleeping-habits/

BOOK, WEBSITE & PODCAST RECOMMENDATIONS

- https://www.youtube.com/watch?v=B7UV35Ek_0I
- https://theplantbasedgrandma.com/plant-based-intermittent-fasting/
- https://www.amazon.com/PlantYou-Ridiculously-Amazingly-Delicious-Plant-Based/dp/0306923041/
- https://www.amazon.com/Vegan-Chinese-Kitchen-Thousand-Year-Old-Tradition/dp/0593139704

REFERENCES

- Prevention. (2024). *Intermittent fasting for women over 50: What to know.* Retrieved from https://www.prevention.com/weight-loss/diets/a61413679/intermittent-fasting-women-over-50/
- Nature. (2024). *Intermittent and periodic fasting, longevity and disease.* Retrieved from https://www.nature.com/articles/s43587-020-00013-3
- WebMD. (2024). *Intermittent fasting for women over 50: What you need to know.* Retrieved from https://www.webmd.com/healthy-aging/what-to-know-about-intermittent-fasting-for-women-after-50
- Harvard Health. (2024). *Is intermittent fasting safe for older adults?.* Retrieved from https://www.health.harvard.edu/staying-healthy/is-intermittent-fasting-safe-for-older-adults
- Intuitive Eating. (2024). *10 principles of intuitive eating.* Retrieved from https://www.intuitiveeating.org/about-us/10-principles-of-intuitive-eating/
- Quora. (2024). *How to handle intermittent fasting when friends and family are not on the same schedule.* Retrieved from https://www.quora.com/How-do-you-handle-intermittent-fasting-when-friends-and-family-are-not-on-the-same-schedule
- Healthline. (2024). *The definitive guide to healthy eating in your 50s and 60s.* Retrieved from https://www.healthline.com/nutrition/healthy-eating-50s-60s
- Medical News Today. (2024). *Menopause: Low-fat vegan diet may help reduce hot flashes.* Retrieved from https://www.medicalnewstoday.com/articles/can-a-vegan-diet-prevent-hot-flashes-at-menopause
- IFM. (2024). *Chrononutrition: Food timing, circadian fasting, and the gut microbiome.* Retrieved from https://www.ifm.org/articles/chrononutrition-food-timing-circadian-fasting
- National Institute on Aging. (2024). *Dietary supplements for older adults.* Retrieved from https://www.nia.nih.gov/health/vitamins-and-supplements/dietary-supplements-older-adults

REFERENCES

- PMC. (2024). *Metabolic disorders in menopause.* Retrieved from https://pmc.ncbi.nlm.nih.gov/articles/PMC9606939/
- Temper. (2024). *Intermittent fasting success story: Fasting after menopause.* Retrieved from https://usetemper.com/learn/intermittent-fasting-success-story-fasting-after-menopause/?srsltid=AfmBOoqSmwv1Bz9fSKdC-wpg9oSn76Rko-DoVSD7PxqfXL52kLPGtZKMU
- Canadian Journal of Cardiology. (2024). *Risks and benefits of intermittent fasting for the aging population.* Retrieved from https://onlinecjc.ca/article/S0828-282X(24)00092-8/fulltext
- News Medical. (2024). *Study reveals brain health benefits of intermittent fasting.* Retrieved from https://www.news-medical.net/news/20240625/Study-reveals-brain-health-benefits-of-intermittent-fasting-and-healthy-diet-plans.aspx
- Time Restricted Eats. (2024). *Intermittent fasting and mindful eating: Combining for optimal health.* Retrieved from https://www.timerestrictedeats.com/fasting-information/the-intersection-of-intermittent-fasting-and-mindful-eating-practices/
- Dr. Ruscio. (2024). *What to know about intermittent fasting for women over 50.* Retrieved from https://drruscio.com/fasting-for-women-over-50/
- StatPearls. (2024). *Management of weight loss plateau.* Retrieved from https://www.ncbi.nlm.nih.gov/books/NBK576400/
- Lifesum. (2024). *How to navigate social situations while fasting.* Retrieved from https://lifesum.com/nutrition-explained/how-to-navigate-social-situations-while-fasting#:~:text=Flex%20your%20fast%20window&text=Say%20you%20have%20a%20date,events%20on%20your%20eating%20days.
- Dummies. (2024). *10 ways to stay motivated when fasting.* Retrieved from https://www.dummies.com/article/body-mind-spirit/physical-health-well-being/diet-nutrition/general-diet-nutrition/10-ways-to-stay-motivated-when-fasting-203870/
- Journal of the Academy of Nutrition and Dietetics. (2024). *A narrative review of intermittent fasting with exercise.* Retrieved from https://www.jandonline.org/article/S2212-2672(24)00254-5/fulltext
- Zero Longevity. (2024). *How to pair mindful eating with mindful fasting.* Retrieved from https://zerolongevity.com/blog/how-to-pair-mindful-eating-with-mindful-fasting/

REFERENCES

- Rebholz, C. M., et al. (2019). "Plant-Based Diets Are Associated With a Lower Risk of Incident Cardiovascular Disease, Cardiovascular Disease Mortality, and All-Cause Mortality in a General Population of Middle-Aged Adults." Journal of the American Heart Association, 8(16), e012865. Retrieved from https://www.ahajournals.org/doi/10.1161/JAHA.119.012865